How to Draw **kawaii** FOR KIDS

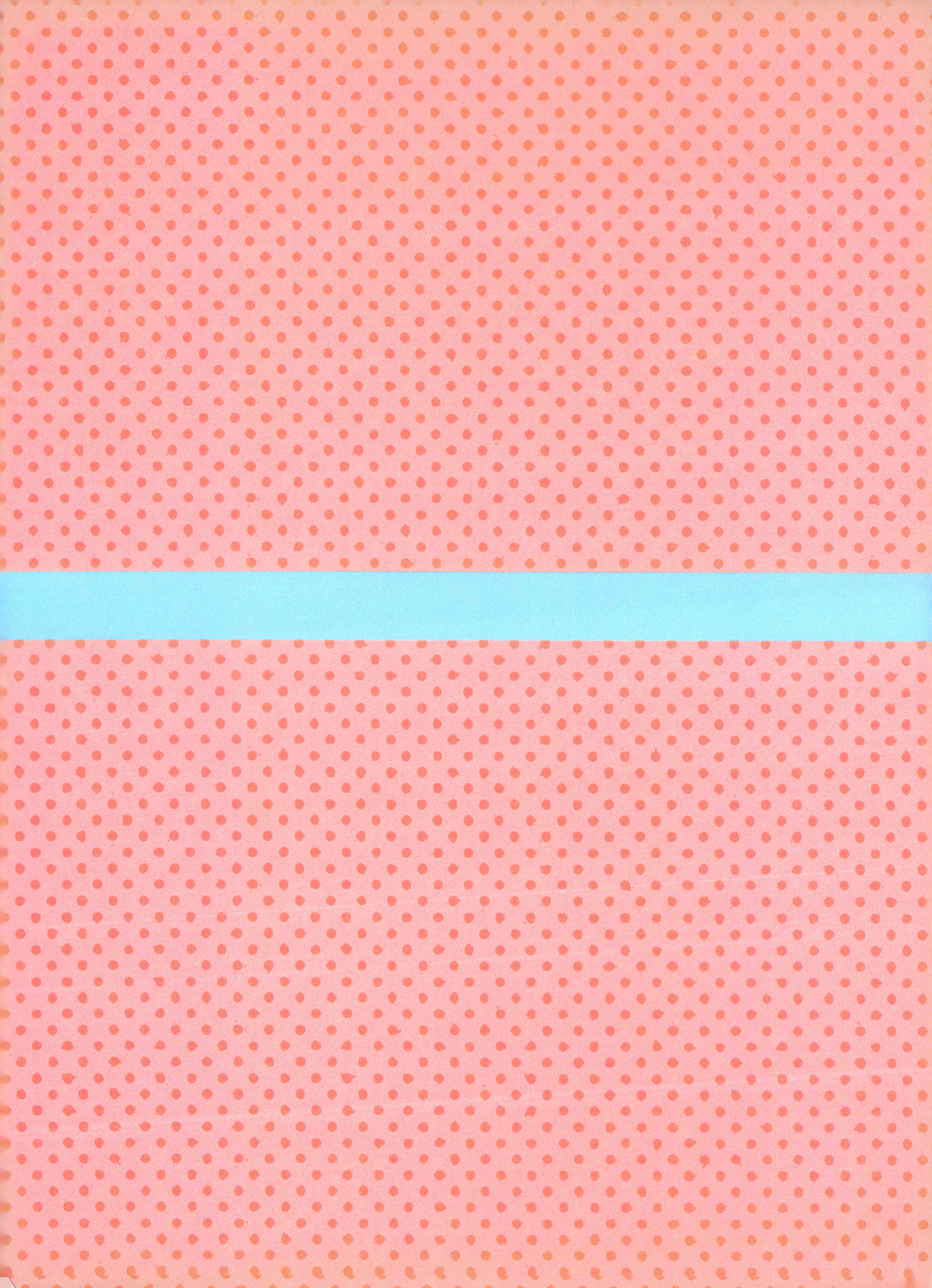

How to Draw kawaii

FOR KIDS A STEP-BY-STEP GUIDE

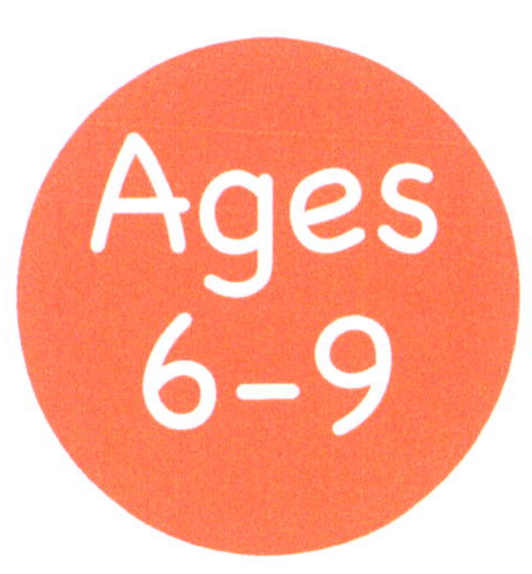

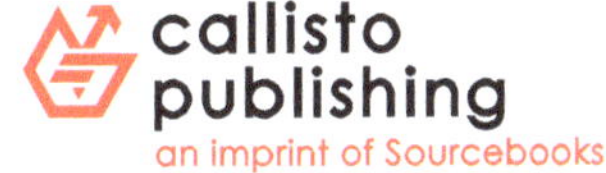

Interior and Cover Designer: Richard Tapp
Art Producer: Megan Baggott
Editor: Lia Brown
Production Editor: Matthew Burnett
Production Manager: Martin Worthington

Published by Callisto Publishing LLC C/O Sourcebooks LLC
P.O. Box 4410, Naperville, Illinois 60567-4410
(630) 961-3900
callistopublishing.com

Printed in the United States of America.

Part 1

Welcome to Drawing Kawaii

Welcome to the wonderful world of drawing kawaii. Kawaii is a Japanese word that means cute. The sweet style can be used to draw animals, people, clothing, and other items.

Drawing can be a lot of fun, especially when the things you're learning to draw are so adorable! Inside this book you will find all the tools you need in order to learn basic important skills and get started.

Everyone can draw, but there's a catch. If you really want to succeed, you will be told by any artist to do one thing: practice, practice, practice. The fact is, the more you do something—anything—the better you will become at it. This doesn't mean you won't hit a few bumps along the way; let's face it, no one is perfect. But if you keep trying, even when things don't work out the first time, you will be able to draw in a way you never dreamed possible.

Drawing is really important. It can help you write, tell stories, share ideas, solve problems, build imagination, and relax after a stressful day. It can even make it easier to remember things! That's because when you draw, you exercise the part of your brain that is connected to memory, which means every time you make a sketch or a doodle, it's like doing jumping jacks for your mind.

So many things you see every day, from the movies you watch to the clothing you wear, began with a drawing. Now it's your turn to dive into drawing—and through kawaii, you can do so in a way that really lets your personality shine through. You never know where your first pencil marks will take you!

How to Use This Book

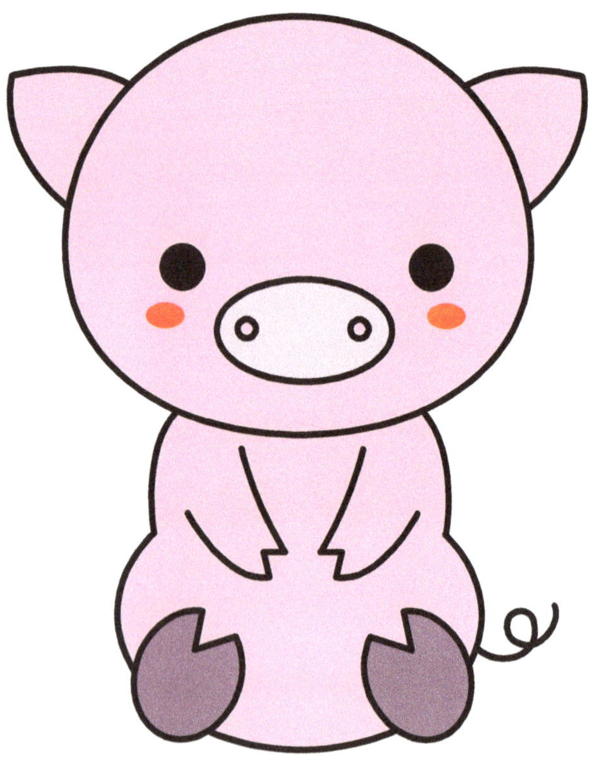

SECTIONS OF THE BOOK

Part 2 of the book is full of drawings, each broken down into six different steps. Look for the red lines to find out where to go next, and if you need to, you can trace over these lines before drawing them on your own. Be on the lookout for the guidelines, which will help you build the image, but should be erased once your drawing is complete.

The next part, "Two-Page Drawings," includes two illustrations of kawaii that require twelve steps each to create. The finished products are a little more complex than the one-page drawings, so they need a few more steps. But don't panic! You are ready for this, especially if you've already tried some of the one-page drawings. Take your time, and have fun.

At the end of the book, you'll get creative! You can trace some of your favorite kawaii characters in the "Try Tracing" section. This will help you get a feel for how all of the lines and shapes fit together to create a finished work of art.

In "Decorated Scenes," you can use the backdrops as a stage for these super-cute characters you have learned to draw. Illustrate the kawaii characters the way they look in the book, or draw them the way you want them to look, and doing whatever you want them to do!

On the very last page, there are drawing prompts to encourage you to grab a pencil and paper and continue your new artistic journey.

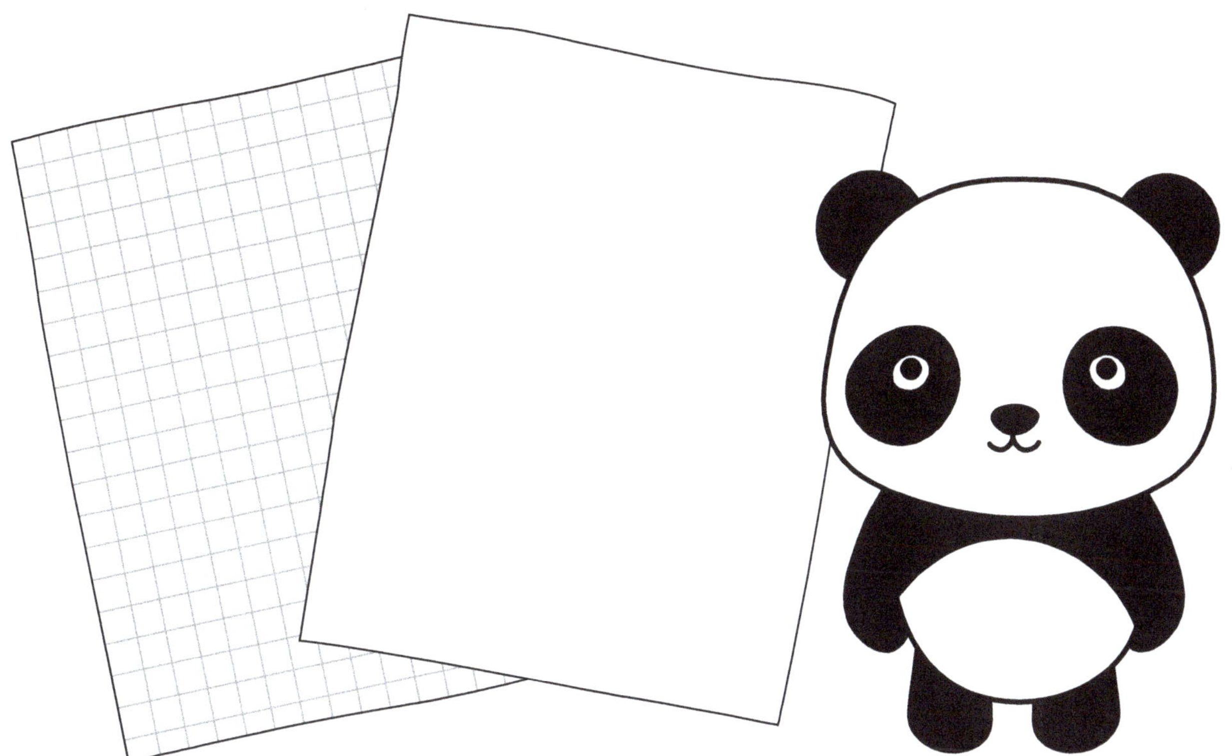

MATERIALS

Before you draw, you will need to gather a few supplies. Pencils, paper, a pencil sharpener, and an eraser are the materials you will need to get started, along with some colored pencils (or crayons) for adding a pop of color.

To begin, use whatever paper you have available. But keep in mind, if you want to work with markers, pens, or paint, you will need thicker paper so your marks don't bleed through. Sketch pads are nice because all your drawings will be together in one place. Graph paper can be helpful for breaking your drawings down into small sections. Thin paper is great for tracing.

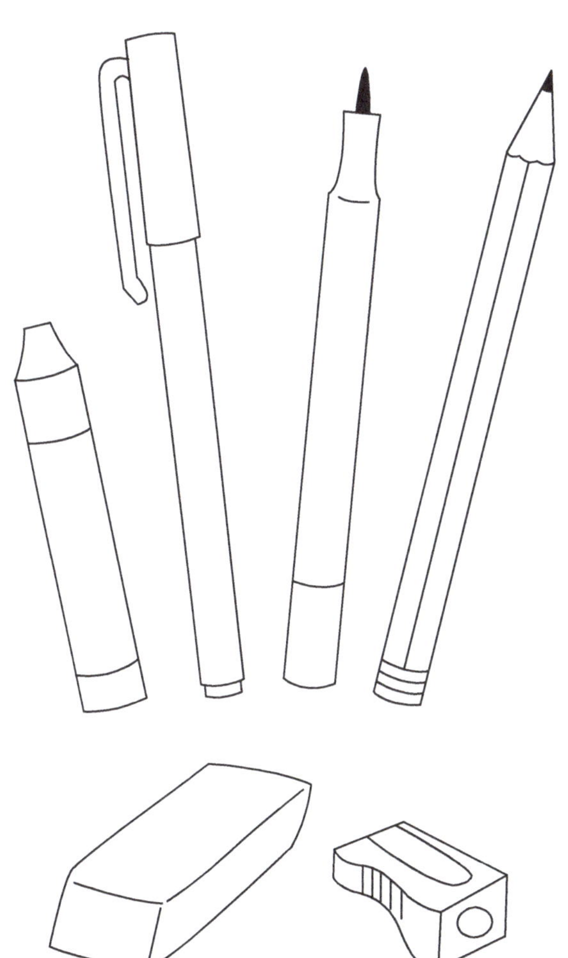

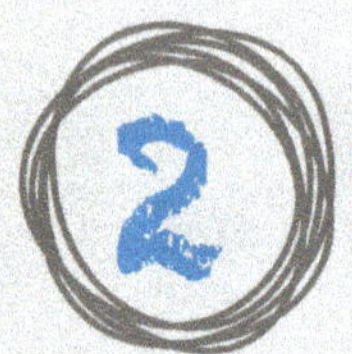

STEP-BY-STEP DRAWING METHOD

Looking at a blank piece of paper can feel really scary. It might even make you say, "I can't draw!" However, when you know exactly where to start, drawing anything—including cute kawaii features and movements—becomes a whole lot easier.

We do most things in life one step at a time. We read books one page at a time, we play games one level at a time, and we build with interlocking blocks one piece at a time. Yet when it comes to drawing, we think we should be able to produce a picture without first breaking it down into manageable chunks.

With a step-by-step drawing method, one line or shape creates a base for the next mark. Drawing kawaii is a great example of this, since many characters, expressions, and objects are made through slight, simple line work. So instead of feeling overwhelmed, you will have the confidence to make your first mark.

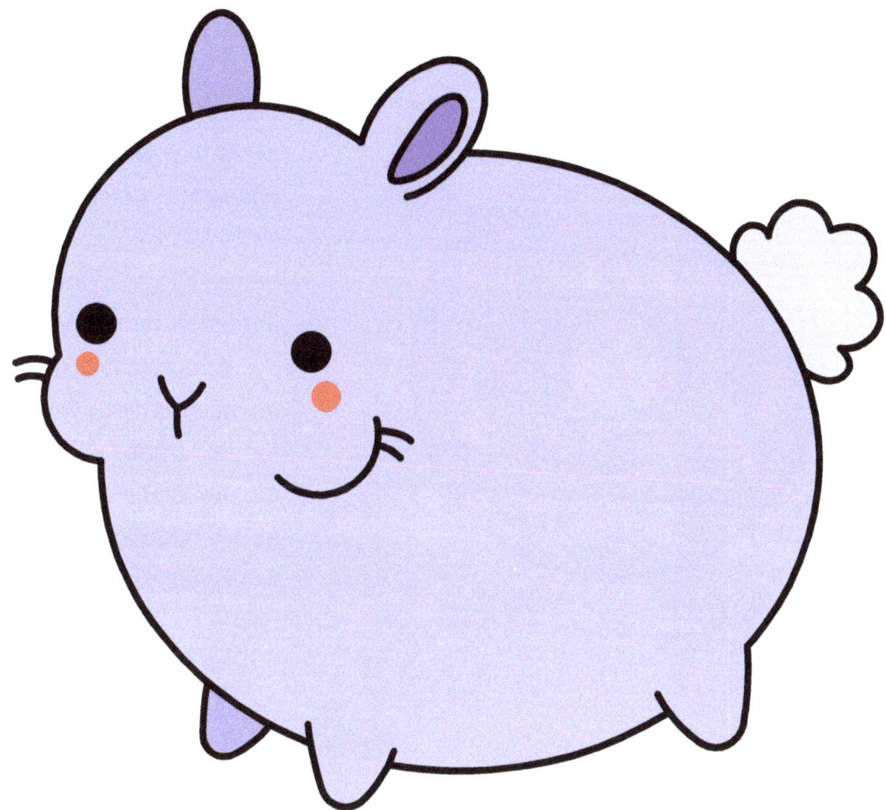

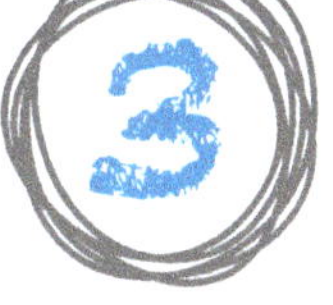

MAKE IT YOUR OWN

Things are about to get interesting, because now you can start to use some of the skills you've already learned to create your own drawings of your favorite kawaii characters and items.

Now that you know that even the most complicated drawings start out with just a few simple lines, you can take any image and break it down into smaller pieces. Begin with a shape, add a line, draw some more shapes, keep adding lines, and so on, until you have a finished work of art.

As soon as you train your eye to find the tiny pieces that make up the whole, you will be well on your way to becoming a line and shape detective who can draw anything. The possibilities are endless, because even the most complicated drawings start out with just one single line.

And remember, if at first you don't succeed, try, try again!

LEARNING TO DRAW SHAPES

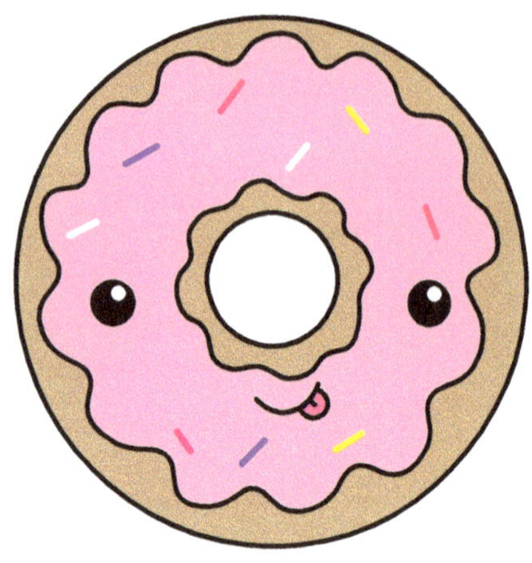

Shapes are flat, enclosed areas with length and width that are created by lines, shaded edges, or changes in color. They can be geometric, with hard sides like a square, circle, and triangle; or they can be organic, with irregular sides like clouds, flowers, and other natural shapes.

If you want to draw something, whether it's an animal, car, monster, or food, you need to first look for the smaller shapes that make up the bigger picture. Once you start doing this, you won't be able to stop, and soon you will begin to see child-like kawaii faces and shapes everywhere you look.

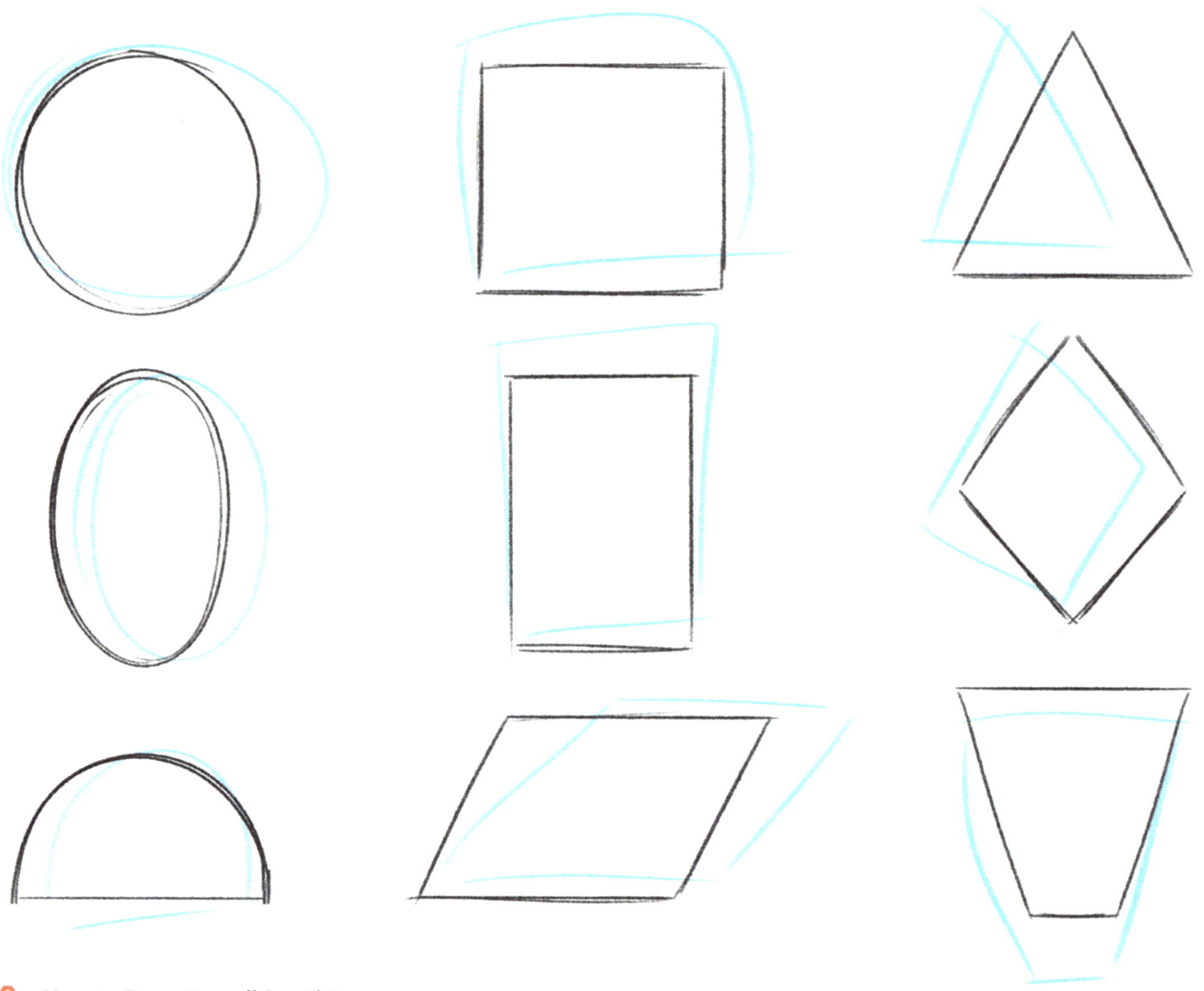

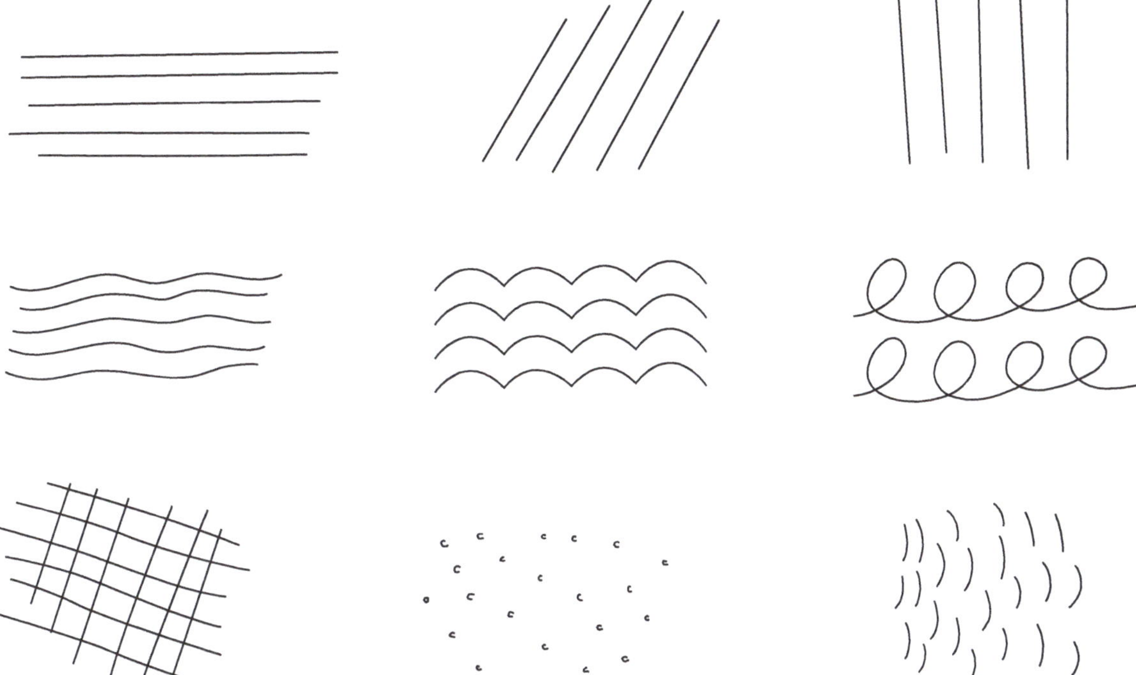

LINES

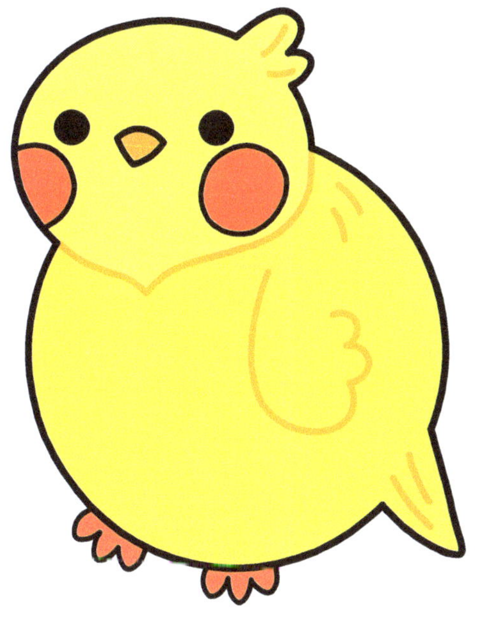

You can't make a drawing without lines, which is why artists love to use them. When looking at drawings, you will notice that lines can be thick or thin, long or short, straight or curvy. They are used to make shapes, create texture, and convey feelings. Kawaii characters are not only adorable, but they're also full of personality. So choosing which lines to use when drawing your favorite characters can be very important.

Horizontal lines run side to side, vertical lines run up and down, and contour lines run along the outside of a shape. In this book, guidelines are used to help build the drawings, but they are designed to be erased. This is why it is really important to work lightly and not press too hard with your pencil.

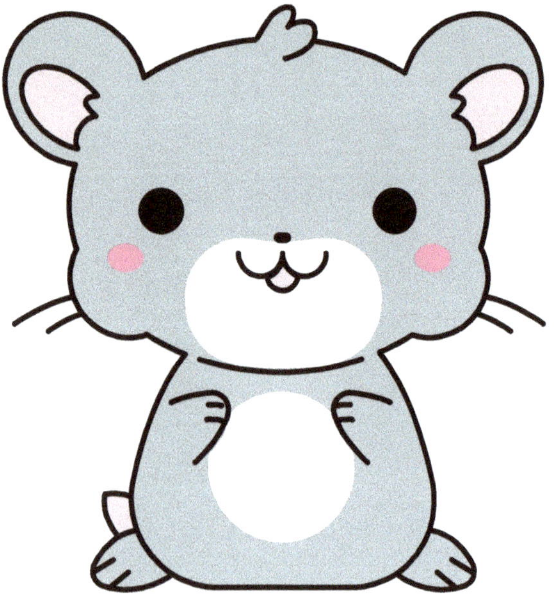

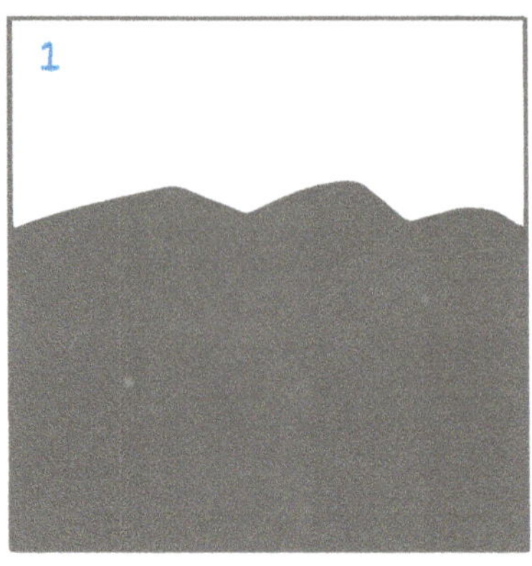

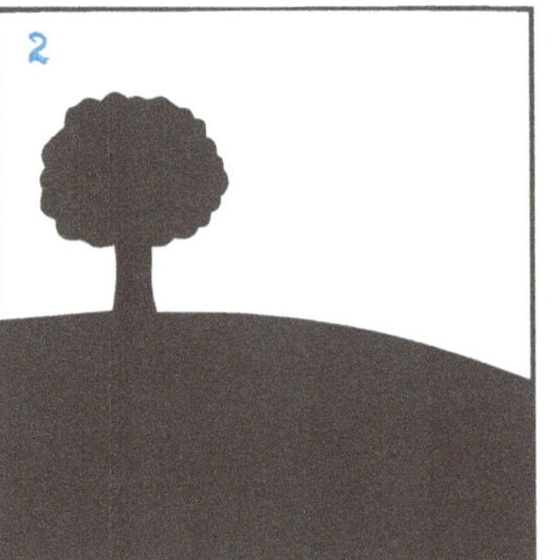

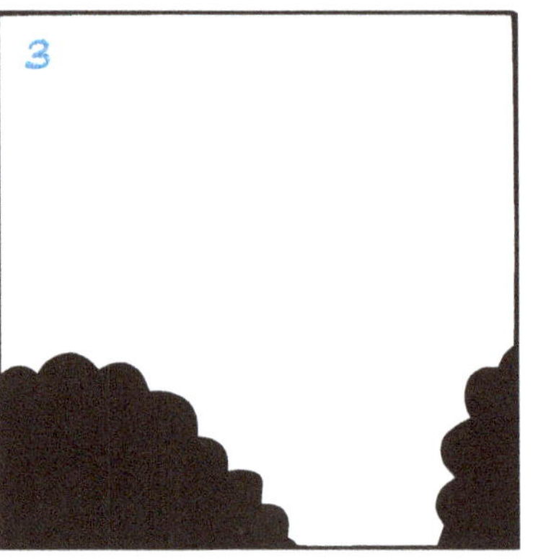

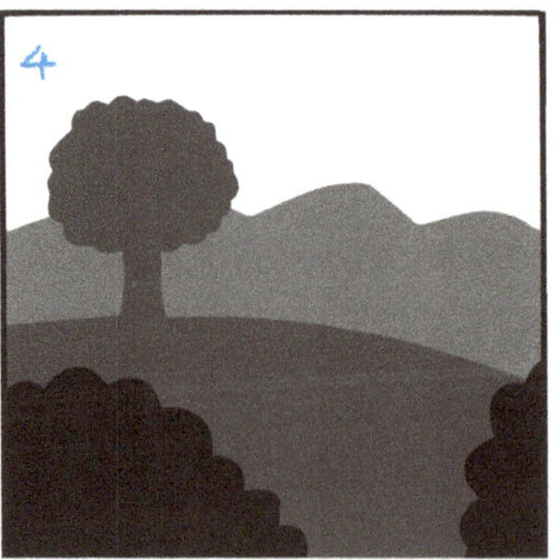

SPACE

You are a three-dimensional being, surrounded by space. Drawings on the other hand, are flat and two-dimensional. However, you can create the illusion of space on a flat piece of paper, by using a few creative tricks.

Overlapping objects in a drawing can create space and make something look like it's farther away than it actually is. The same effect can be created by making items different sizes. For example, a small tree drawn in the background will look as though it is farther away from the viewer than a large tree in the foreground.

Fun fact: The area around an object is known as negative space.

FORM

You've learned that shapes are flat and have length and width. Form adds depth to shapes and is used in a drawing to make something appear three-dimensional, as though it could jump off the page.

Sculptures and other three-dimensional objects have form naturally, but to create the illusion of form (or depth) on a flat piece of paper, we need to get creative. We can use an imaginary light source combined with shading techniques to create the illusion of form in a drawing. Line variations, changes in color, and other visual tricks can also help make something appear three-dimensional.

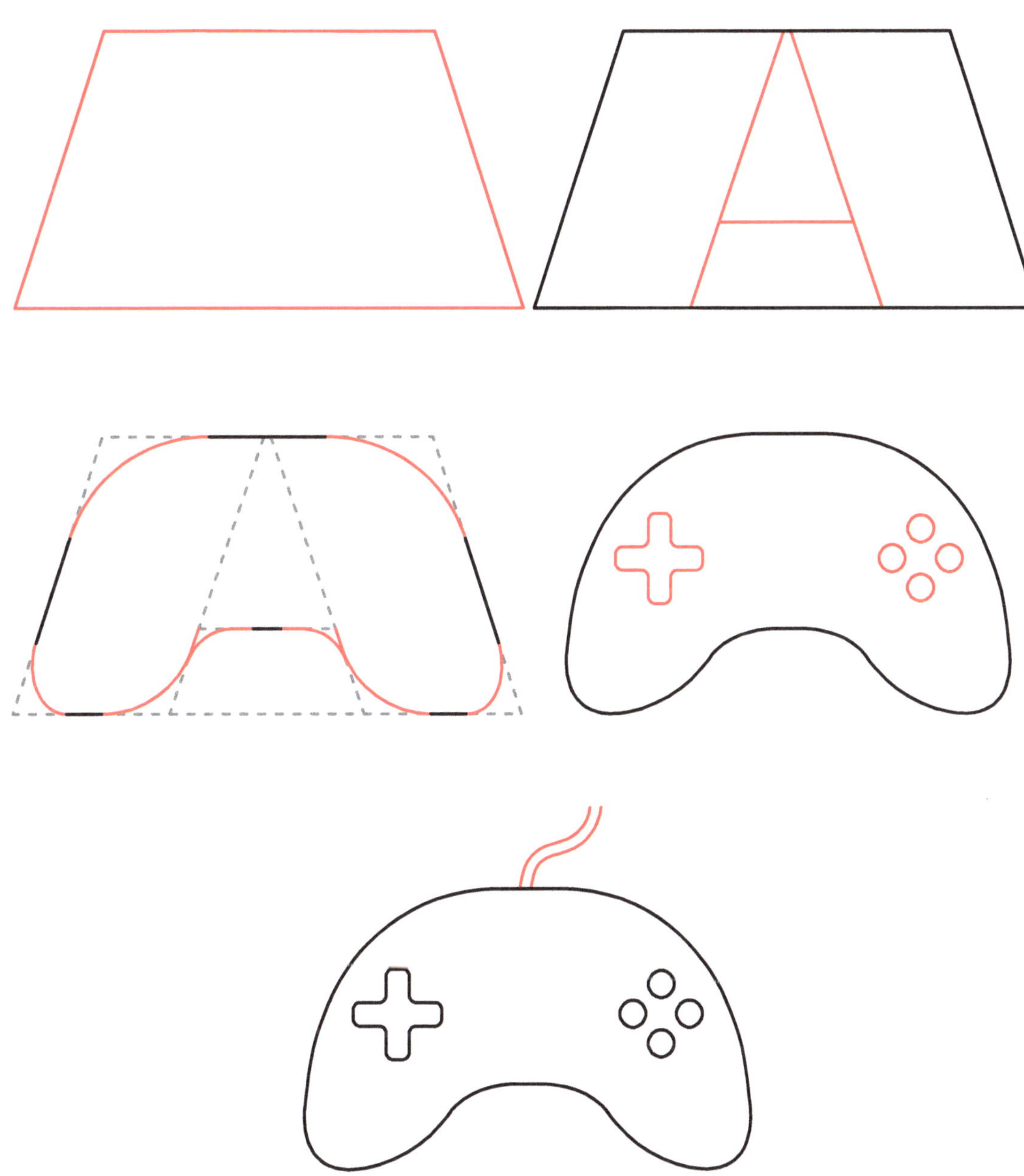

BALANCE

Balance in a drawing refers to how the objects on the page are placed and whether or not the picture looks symmetrical (meaning even, or the same) or asymmetrical (meaning uneven, or different). People generally like looking at things that are symmetrical because they feel balanced and comfortable. But if you want to create more emotion in a drawing, make sure you add a few things to make your picture look a little off-center or unbalanced.

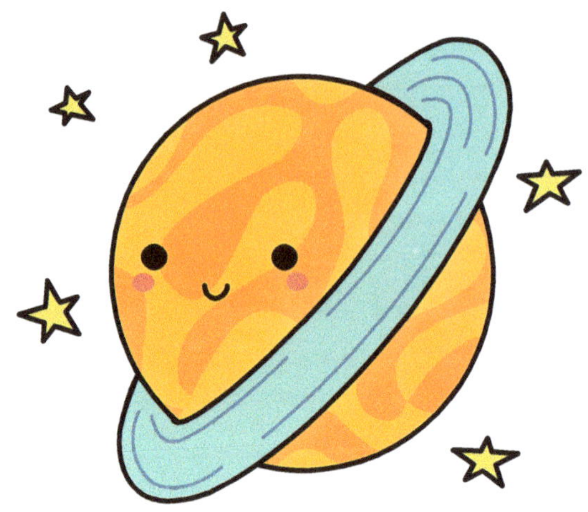

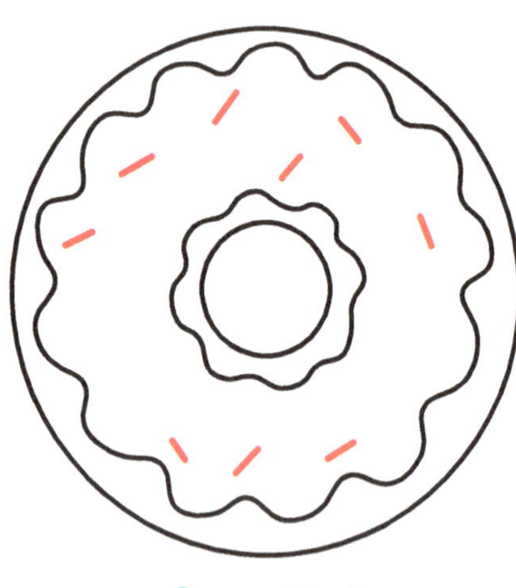

Symmetrical

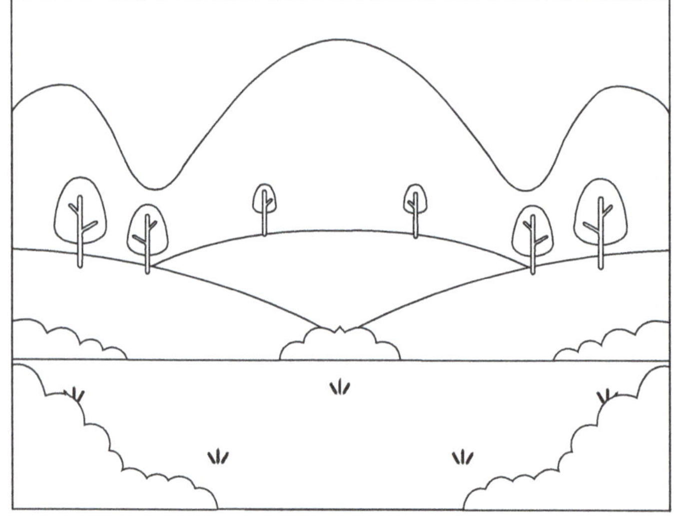

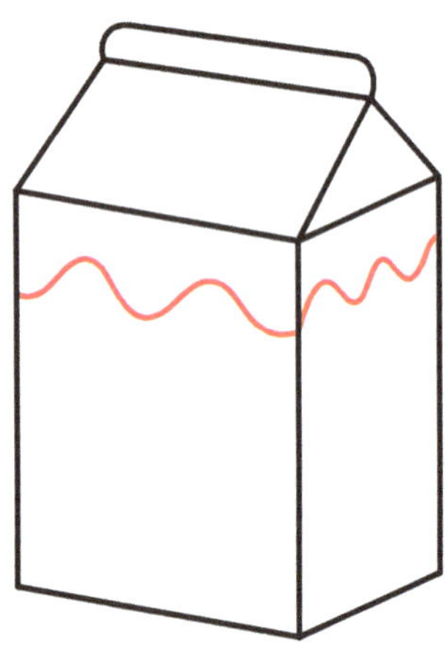

Asymmetrical

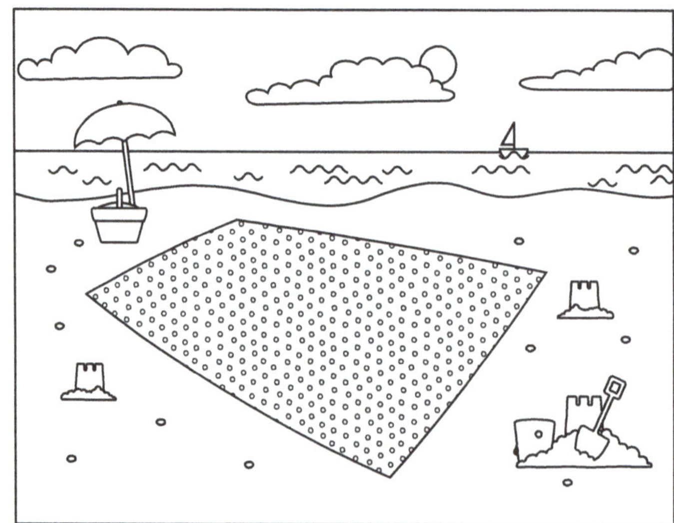

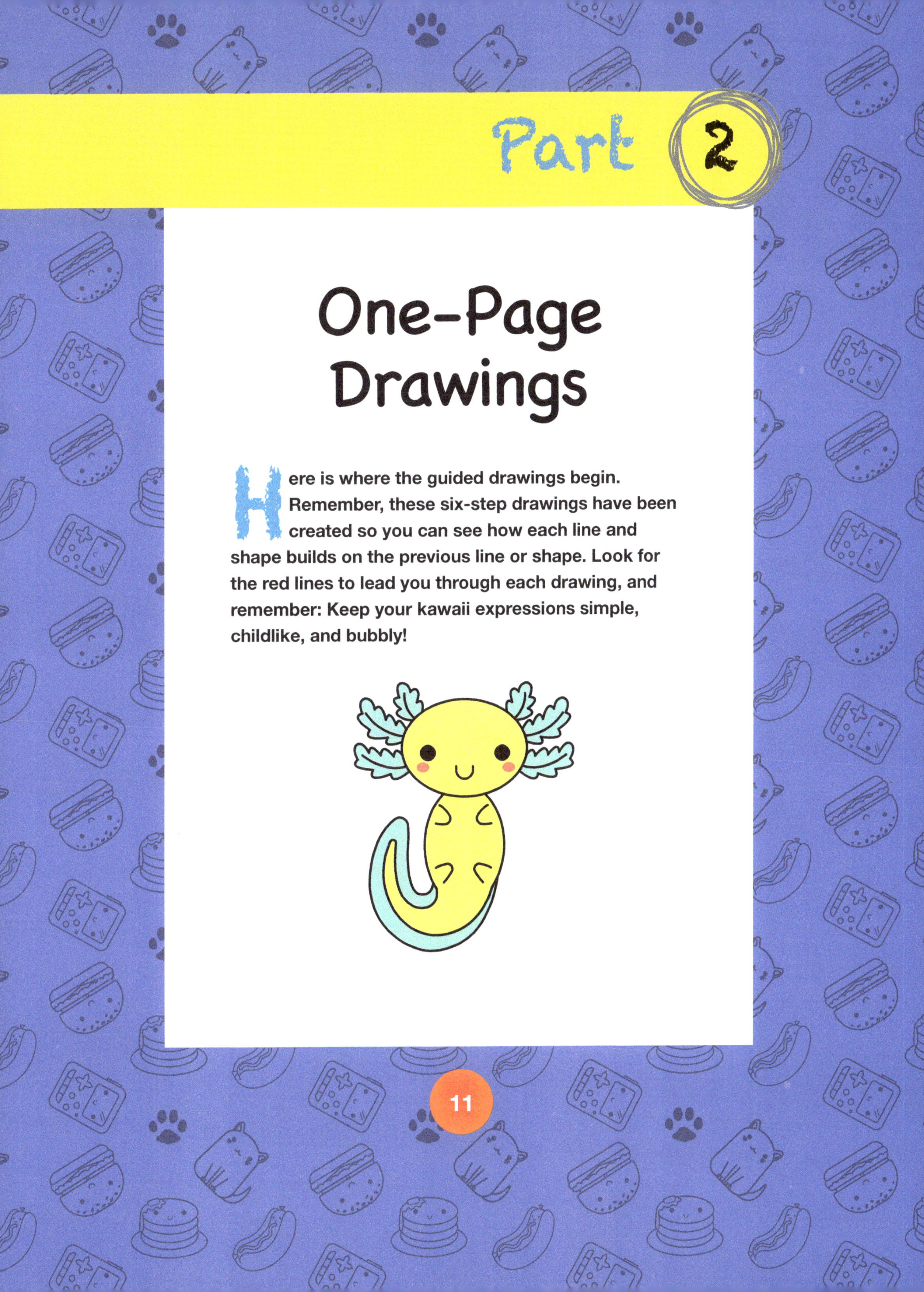

Part 2

One-Page Drawings

Here is where the guided drawings begin. Remember, these six-step drawings have been created so you can see how each line and shape builds on the previous line or shape. Look for the red lines to lead you through each drawing, and remember: Keep your kawaii expressions simple, childlike, and bubbly!

COTTON CANDY CUTE

Create a cloud of sweetness!

1
2
3
Add a peak.
4
Connect the lines with rounded shapes.
5
6
So sweet!

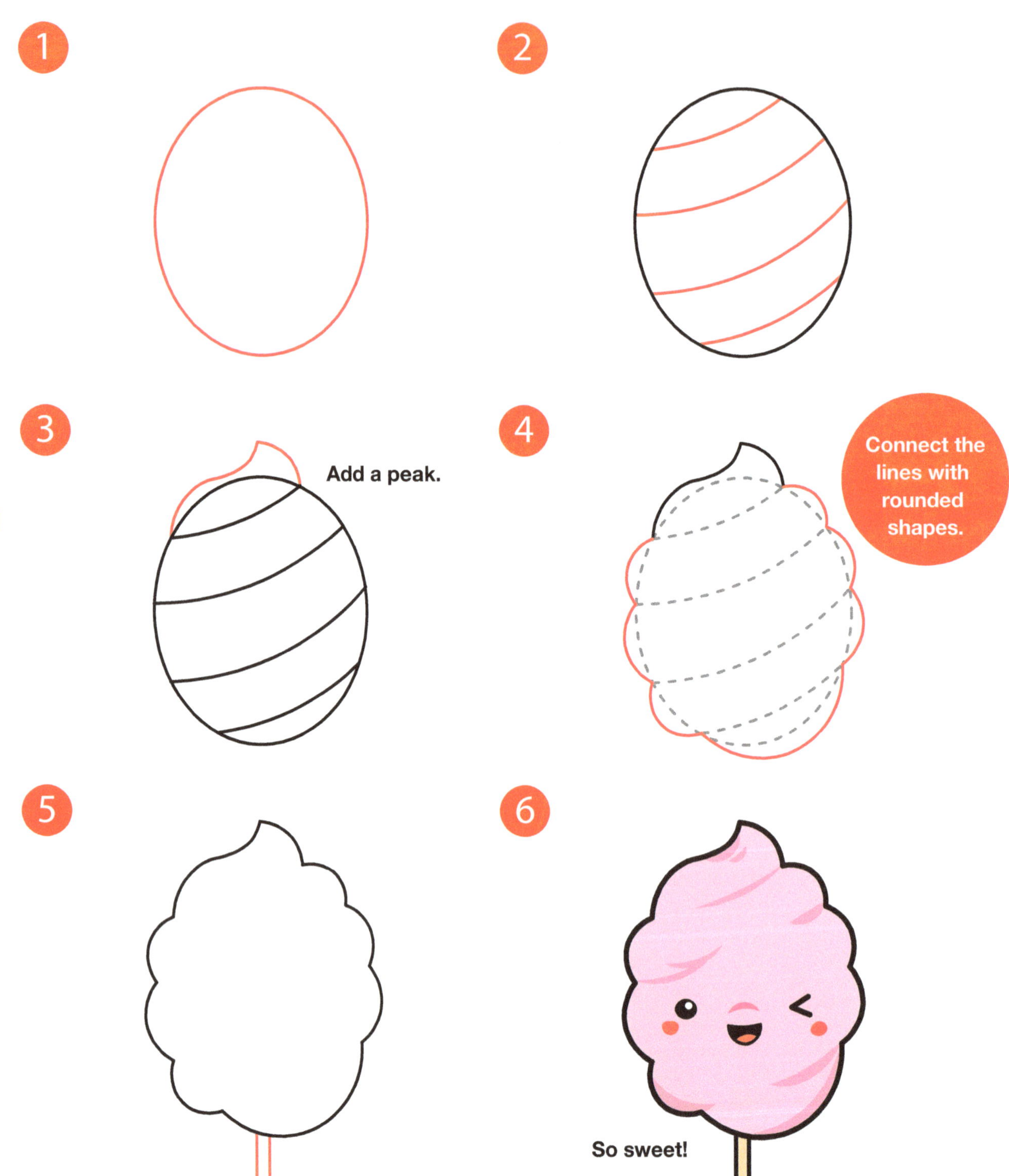

PERFECT PLANET

Draw something that's out of this world!

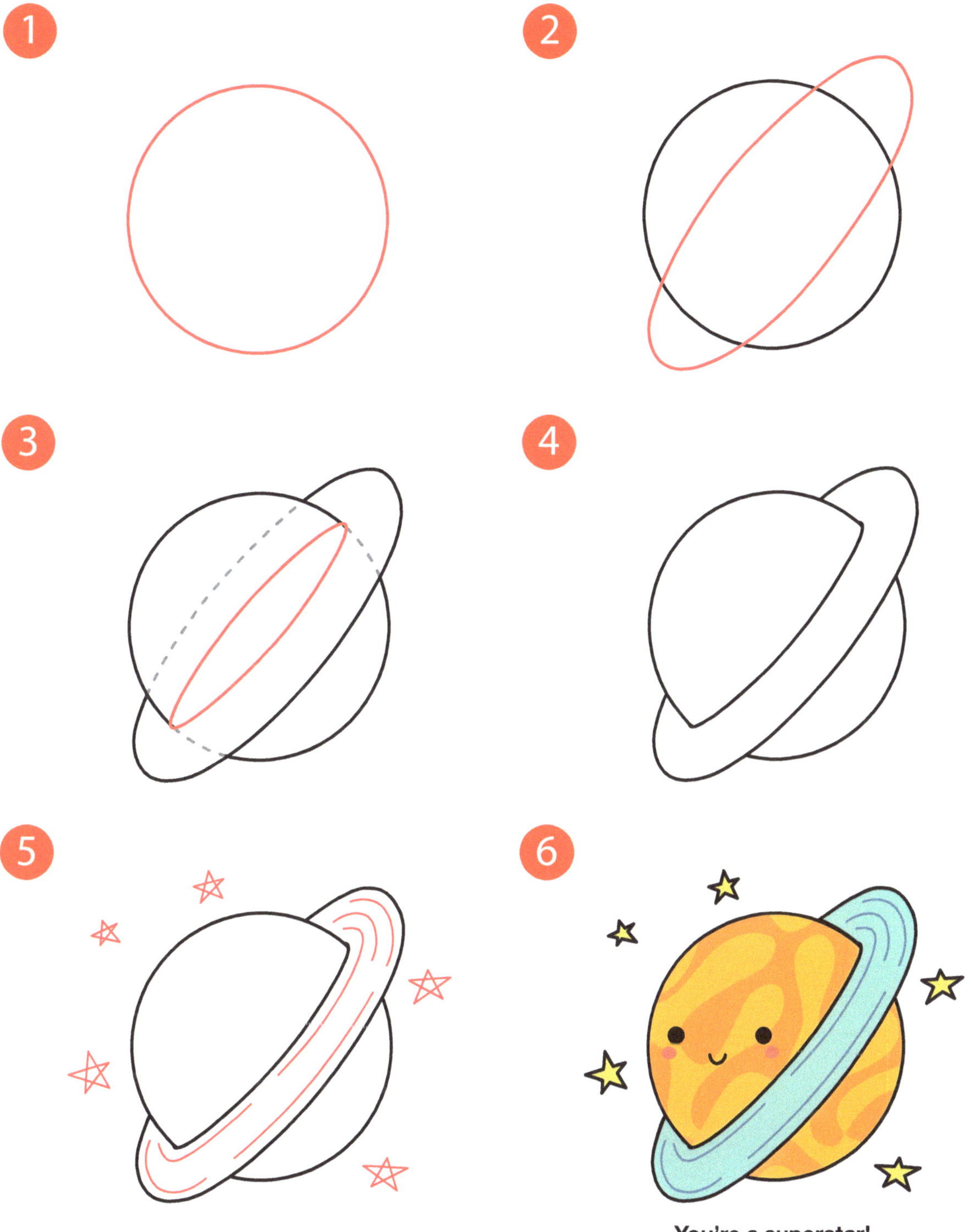

You're a superstar!

DONUT DELIGHT

Keep it sweet with kawaii donuts!

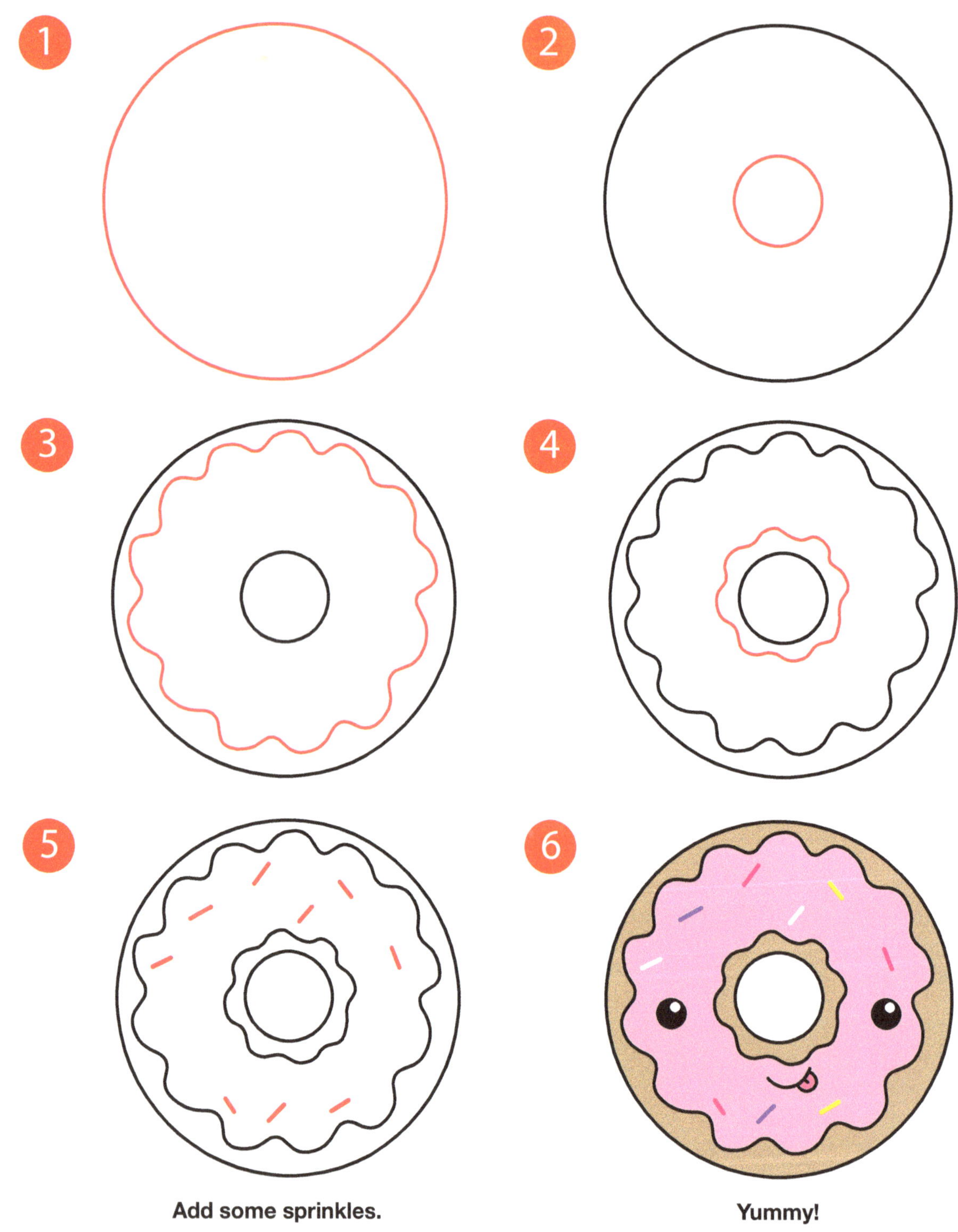

Add some sprinkles.

Yummy!

ADORABLE DINOSAUR

Draw a cute and chubby T-rex!

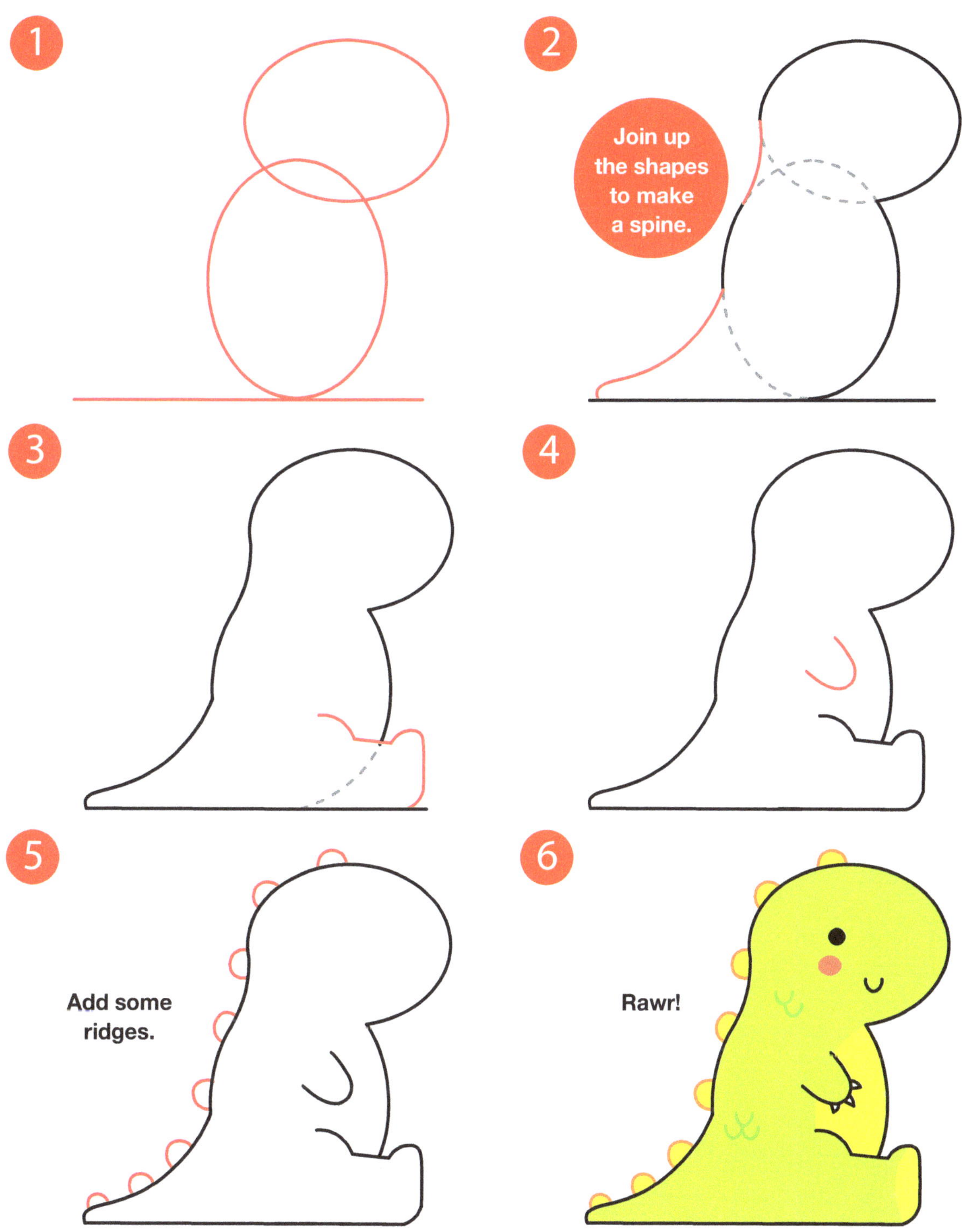

DELICIOUS DUMPLINGS

Draw a whole gang of steamed dumplings!

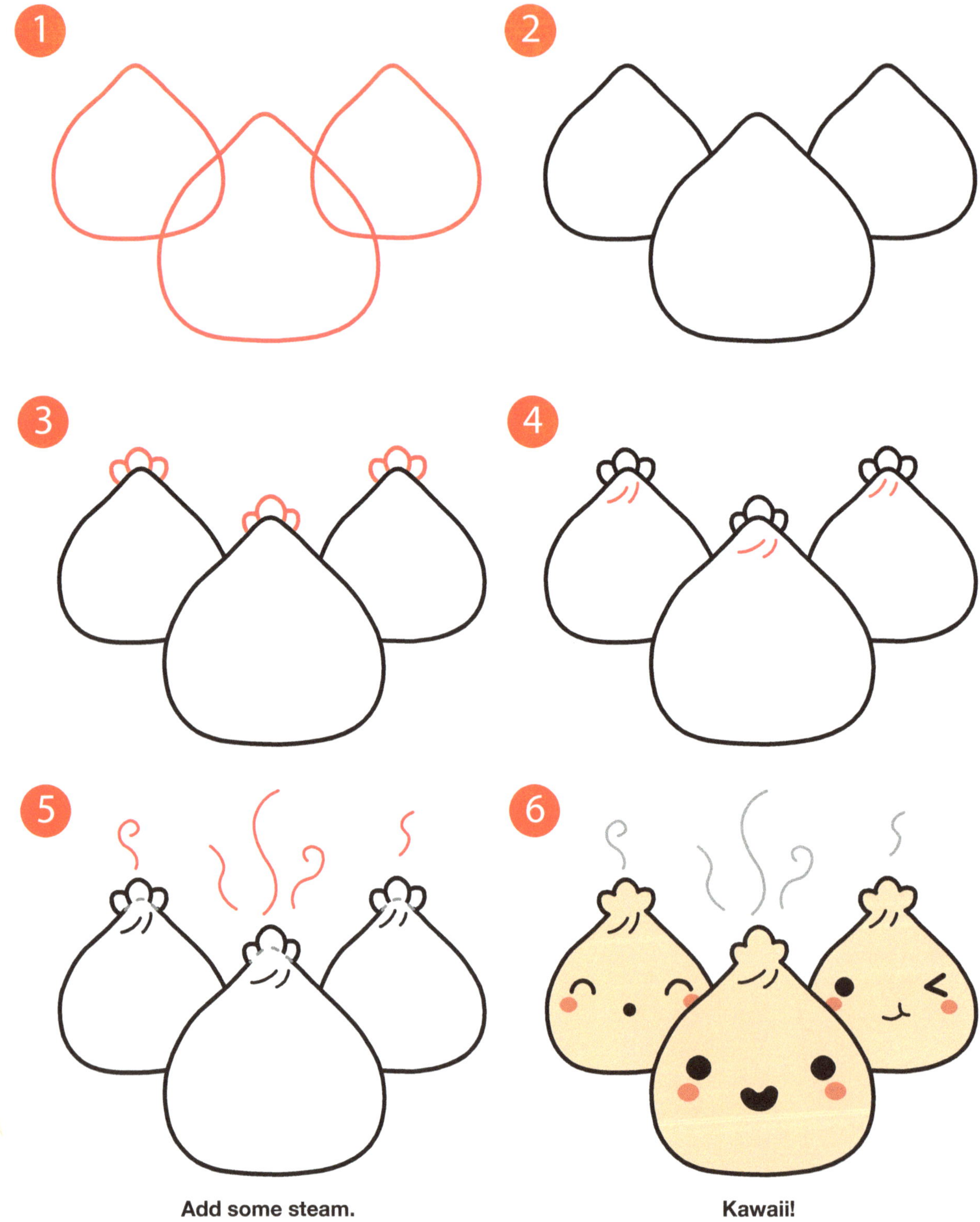

Add some steam.

Kawaii!

COCKATOO KAWAII!

Draw a super sweet tweeter!

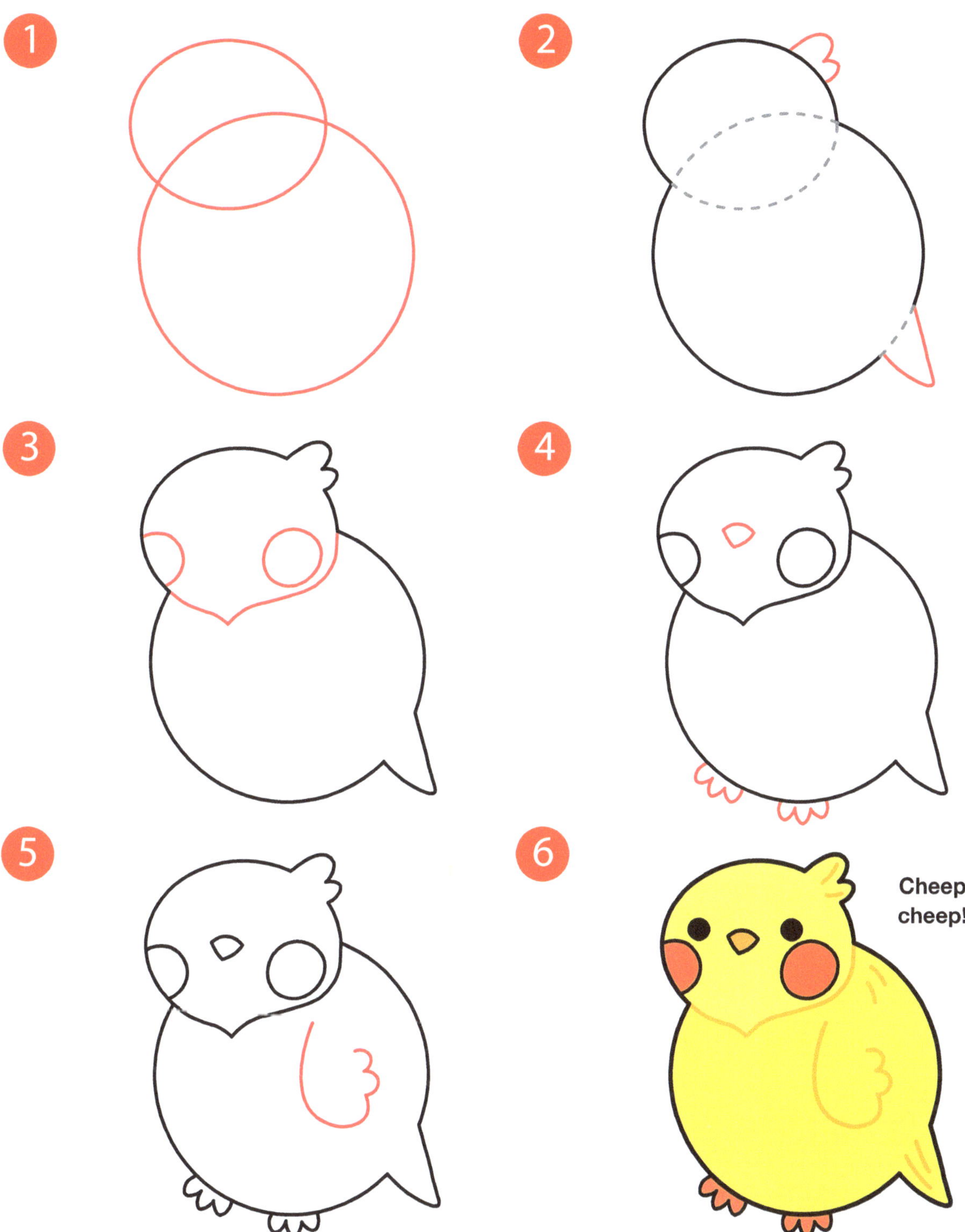

SUPER SUSHI!

You're on a roll! Time for a sushi snack.

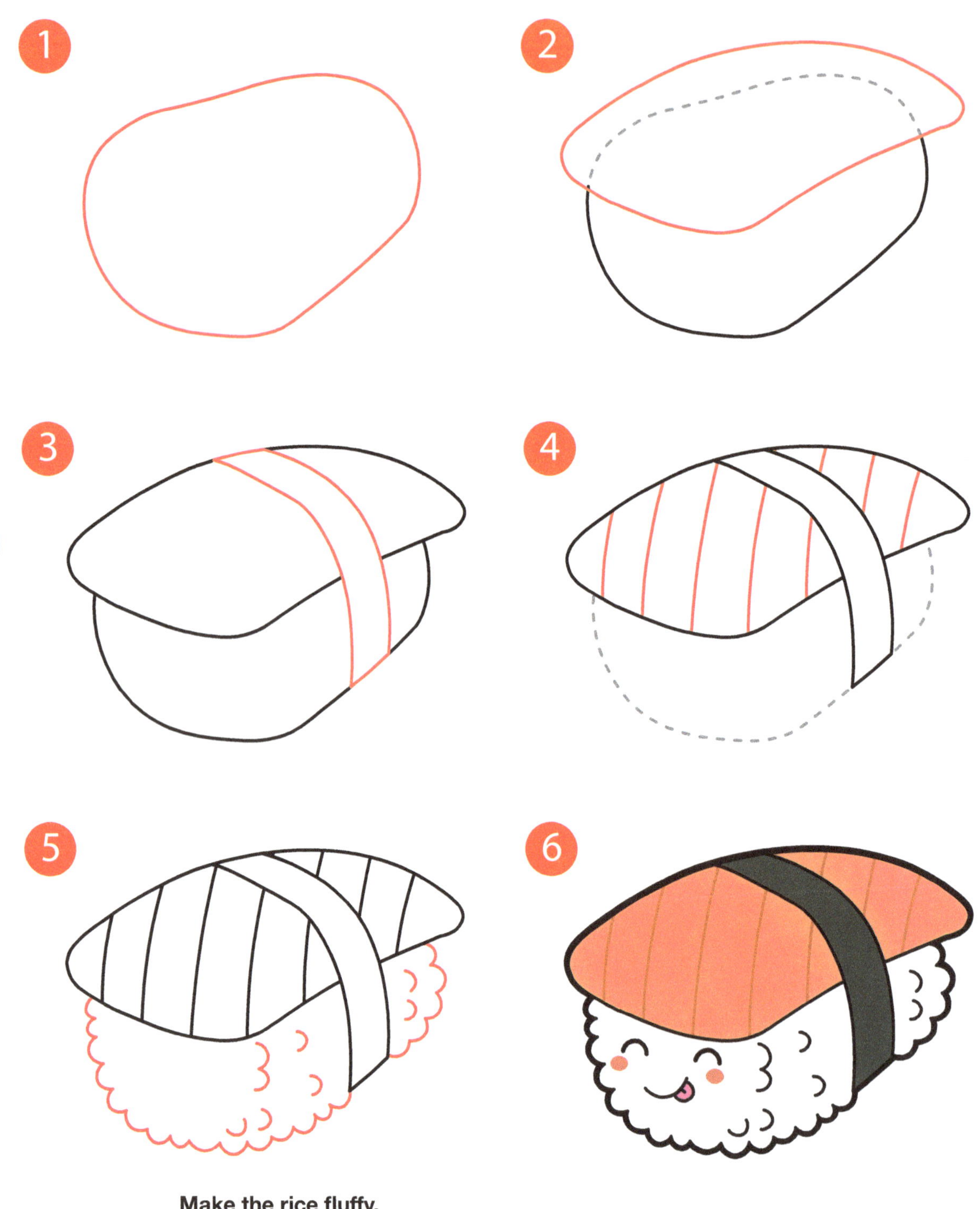

Make the rice fluffy.

PRETTIEST PANDA

Make a super fuzzy friend!

1
2
3
Add ears.
4
Remember the arms and legs.
5
Draw the markings.
6
Now draw me some bamboo shoots!

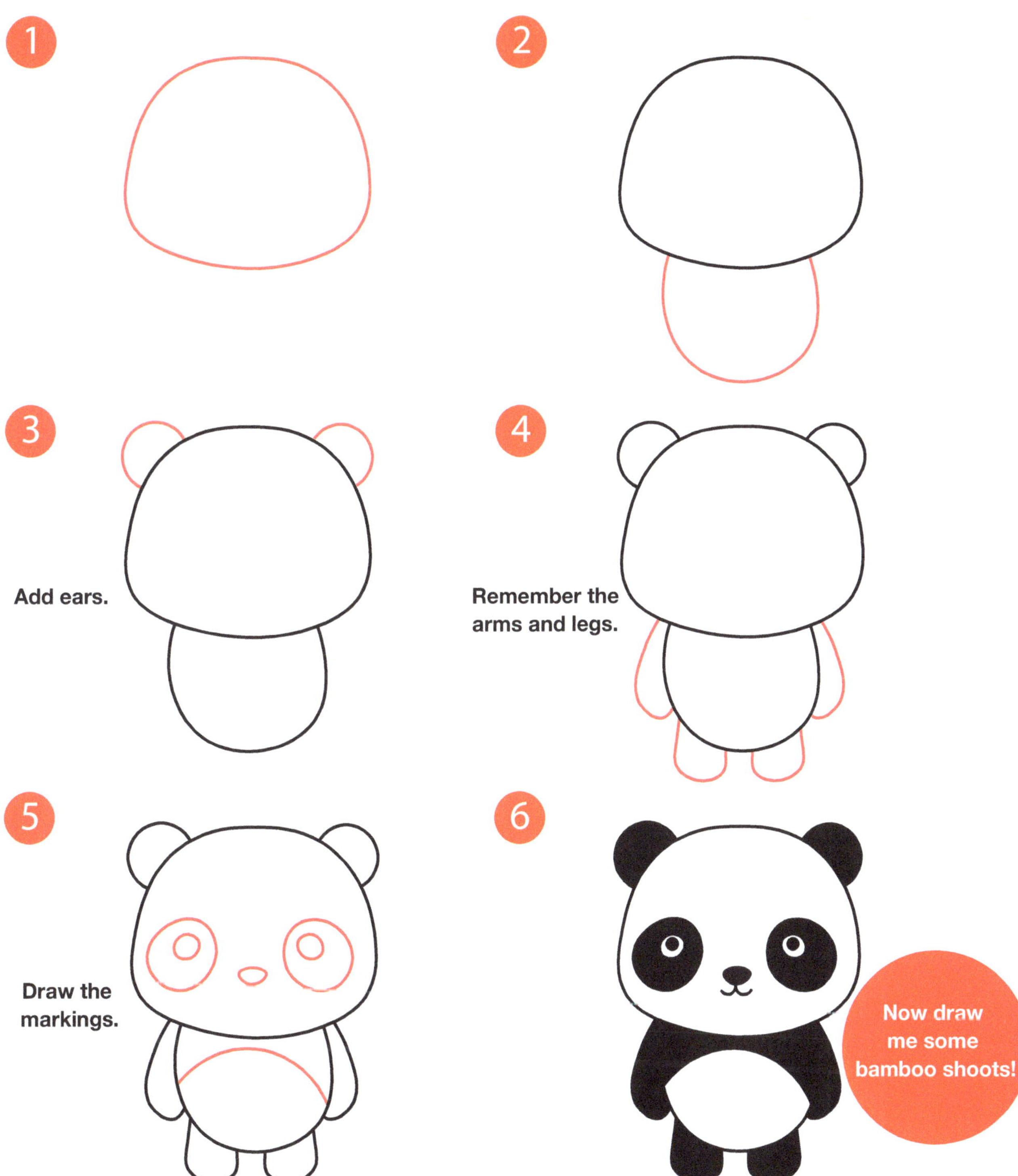

MILK CARTON MAGIC

What's your favorite flavor of milk?

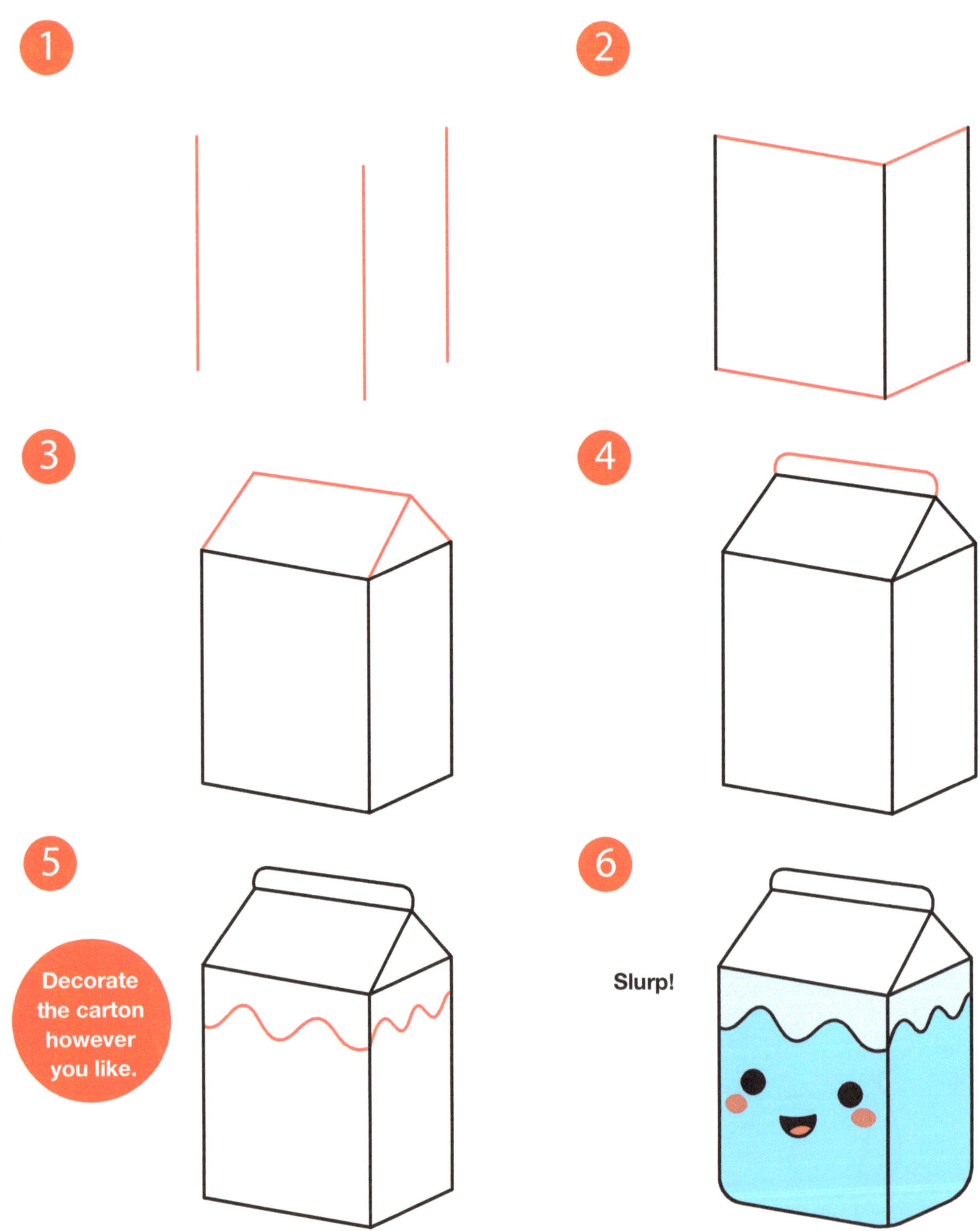

KAWAII KITTY

Meow! Create a cute cat and give it a name.

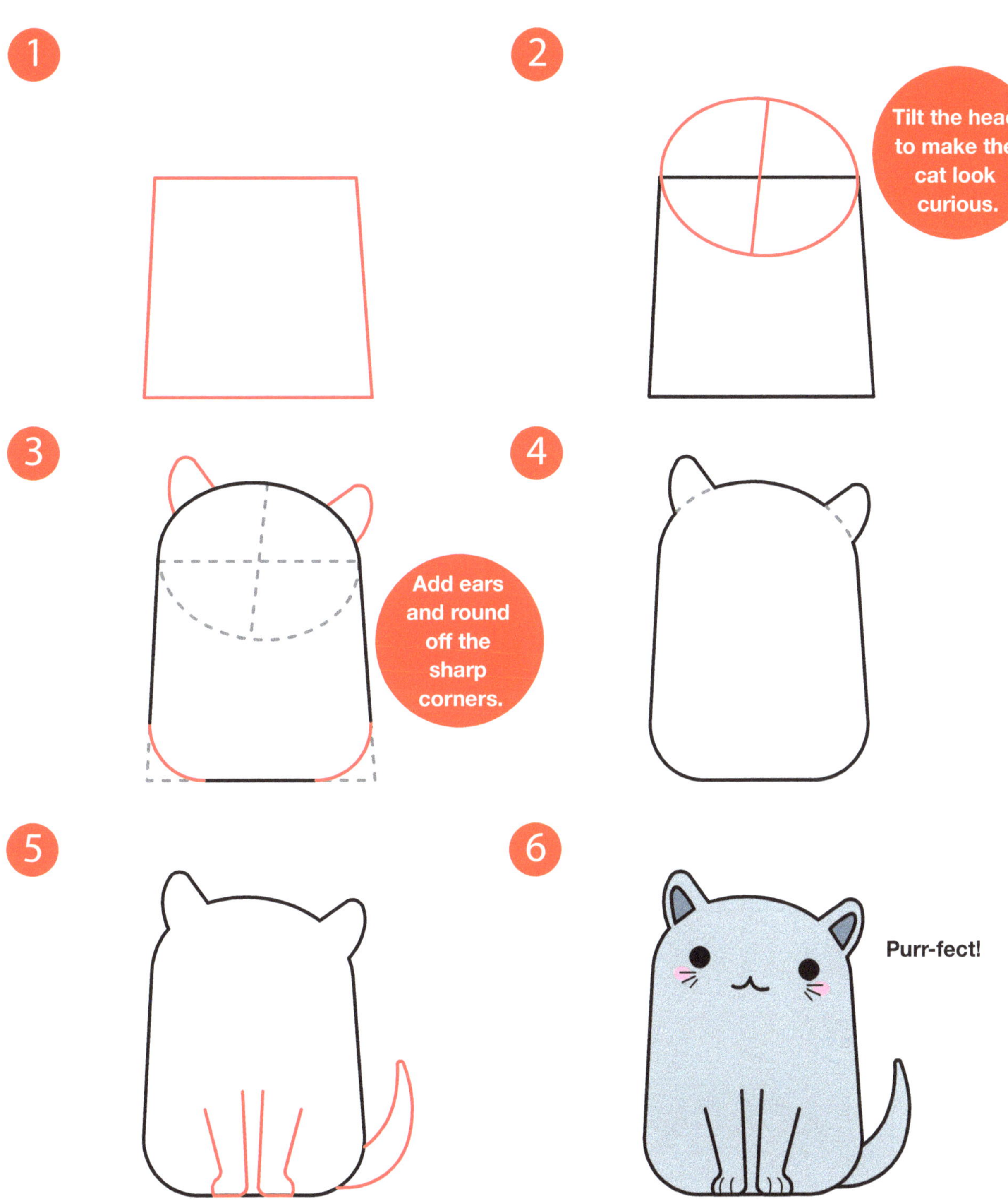

CUTIE CONTROLLER

Draw two for multiplayer mode!

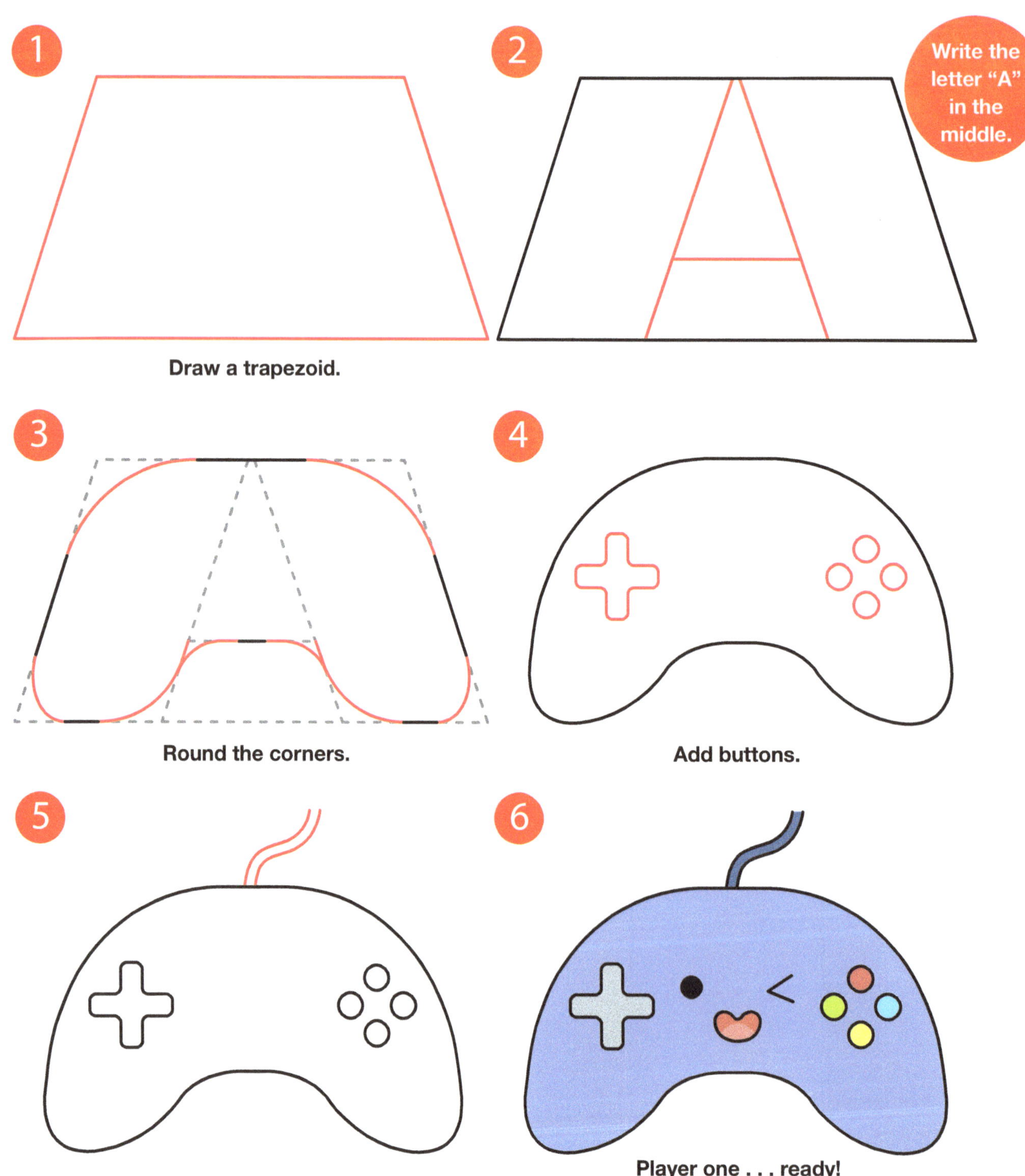

Draw a trapezoid.

Round the corners.

Add buttons.

Player one . . . ready!

ASK A LITTLE AXOLOTL

Draw a super smiley sea creature.

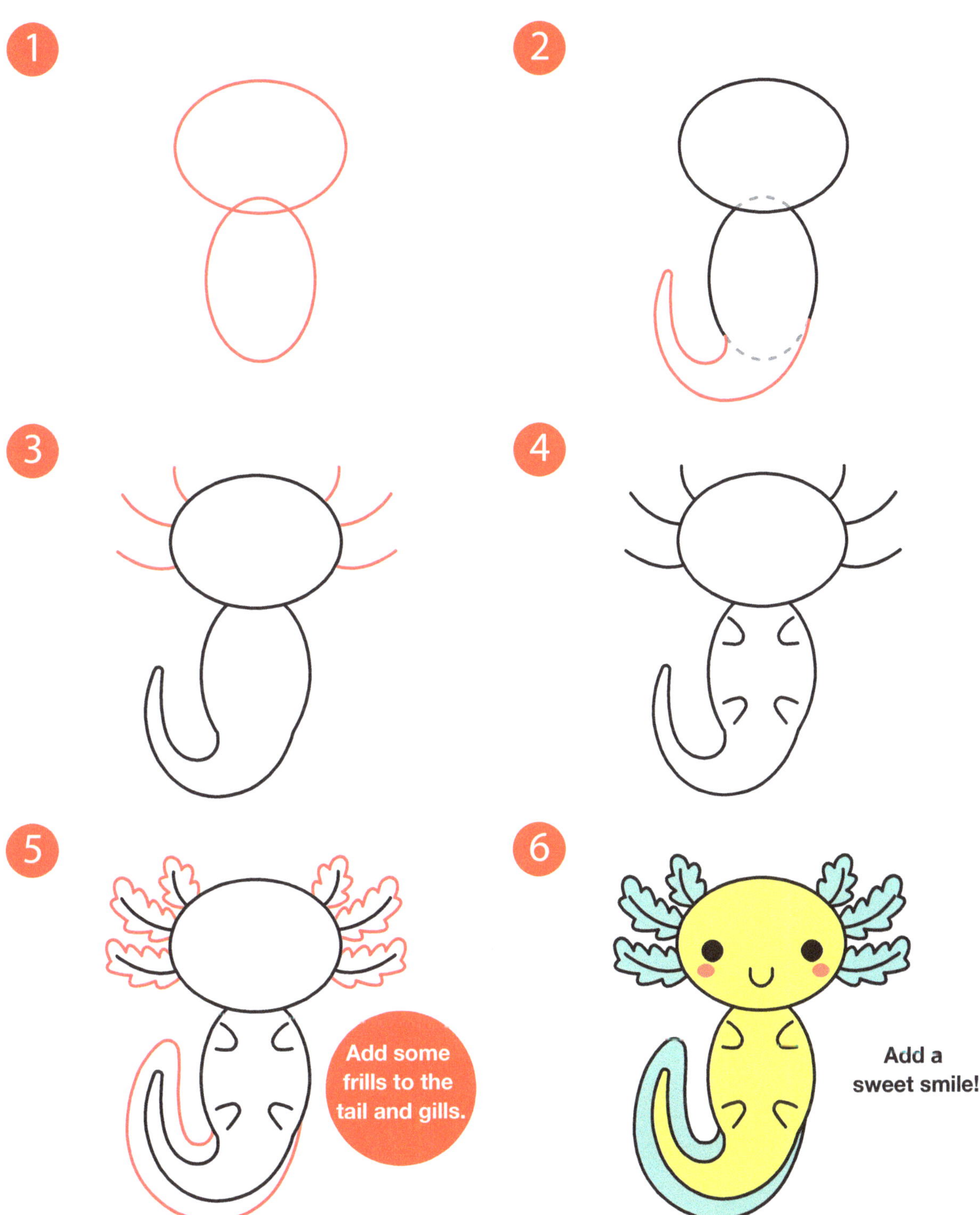

SOMETHING S'MORE

Get cozy round the campfire with kawaii treats!

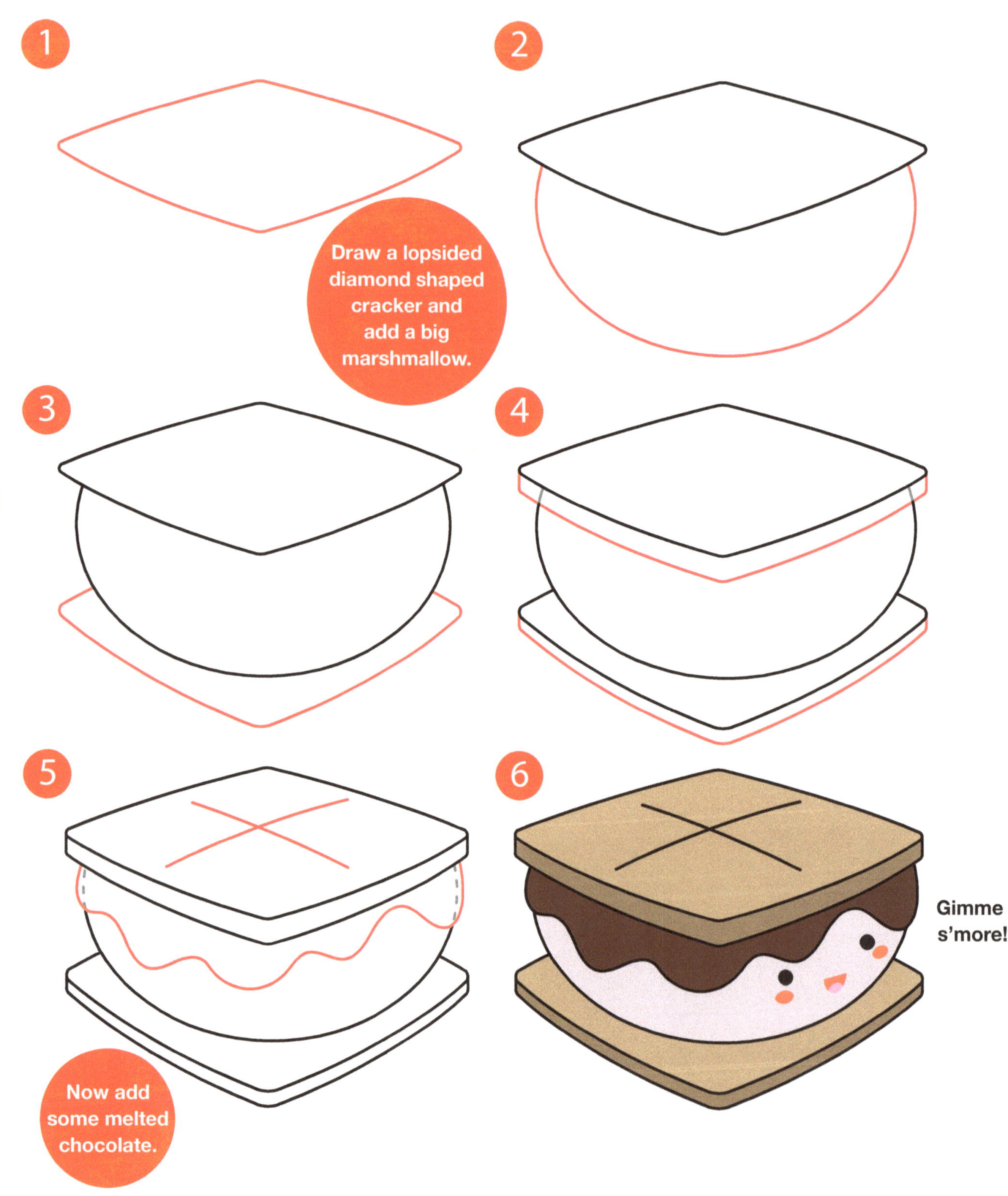

RAINBOW CLOUDS

Make a colorful couple of kawaii clouds!

1
2
3
4
How many colors does your rainbow have?
5
6
Add some raindrops.
It's so beautiful!

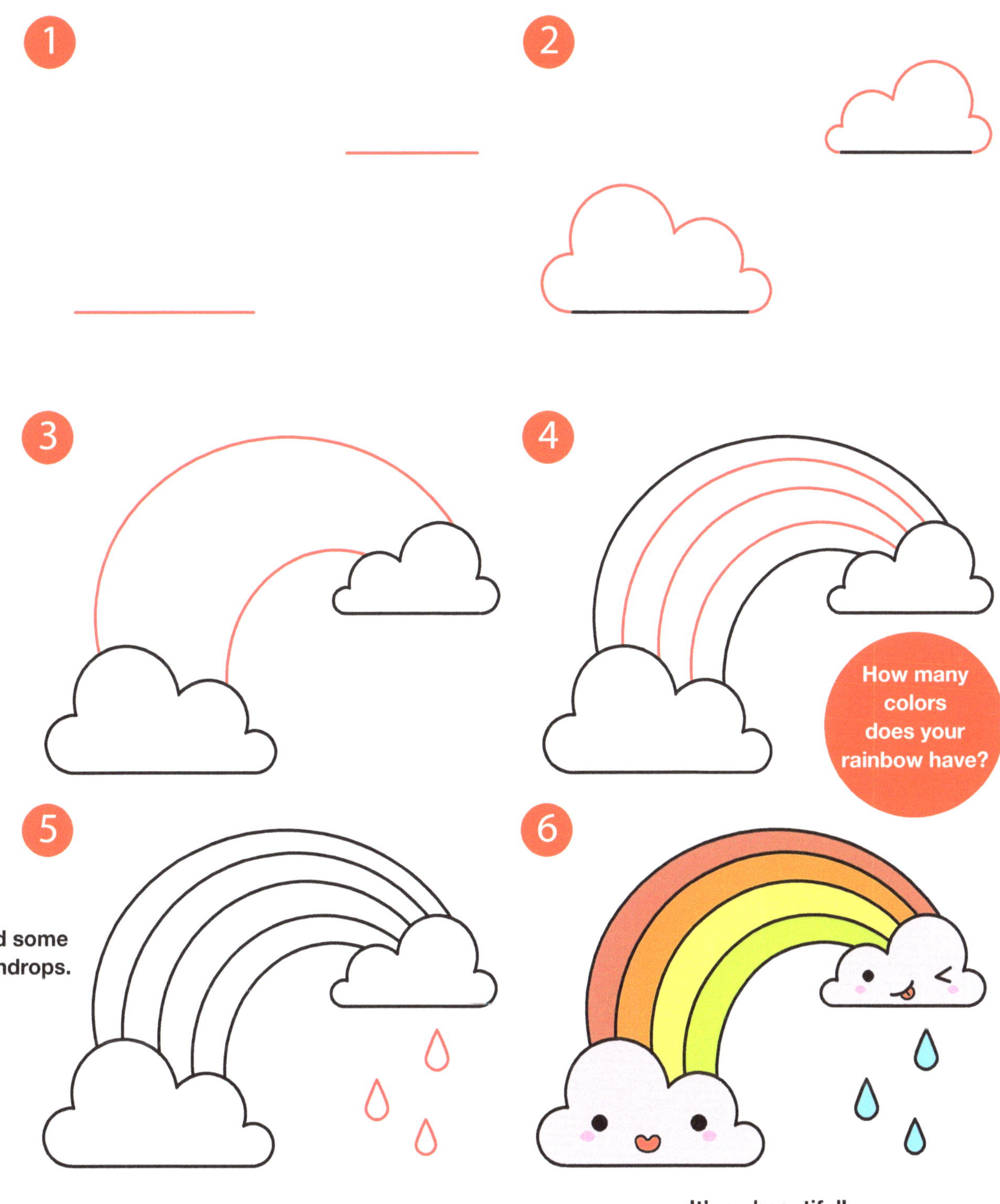

BOUNCING BUNNY

Follow the steps to draw a chubby bunny.

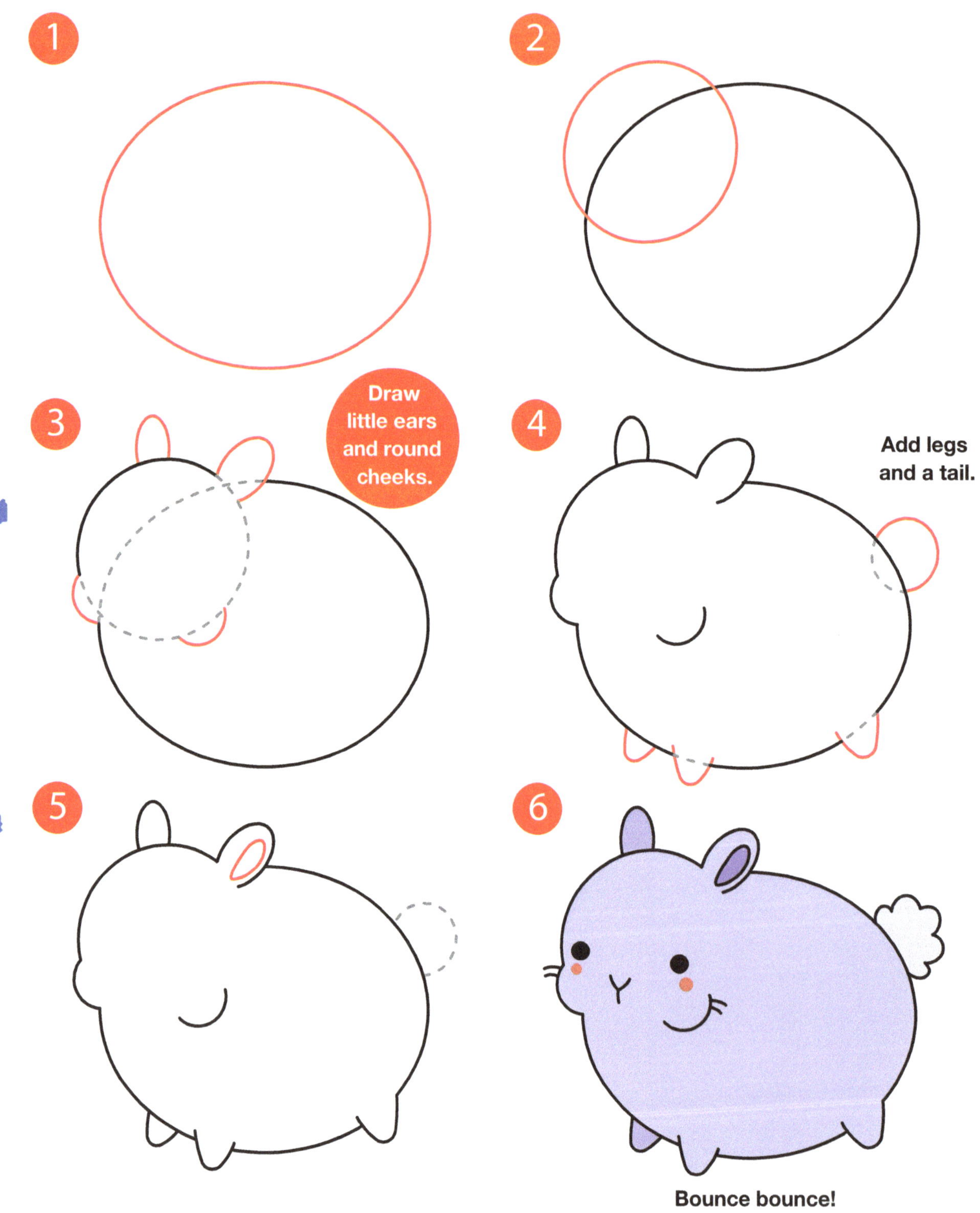

Bounce bounce!

TASTY TACO

Fill it up with your favorite taco toppings!

1

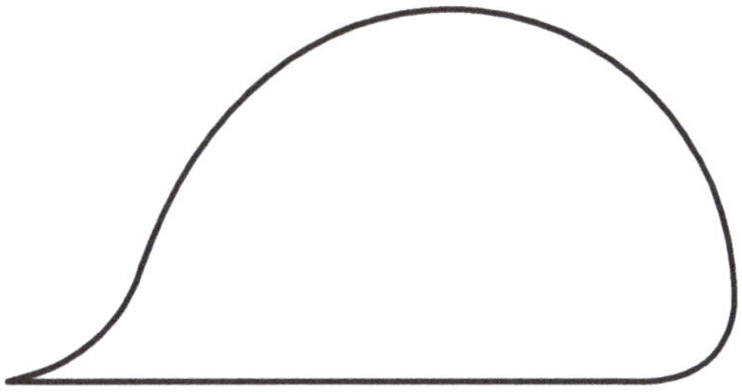

2

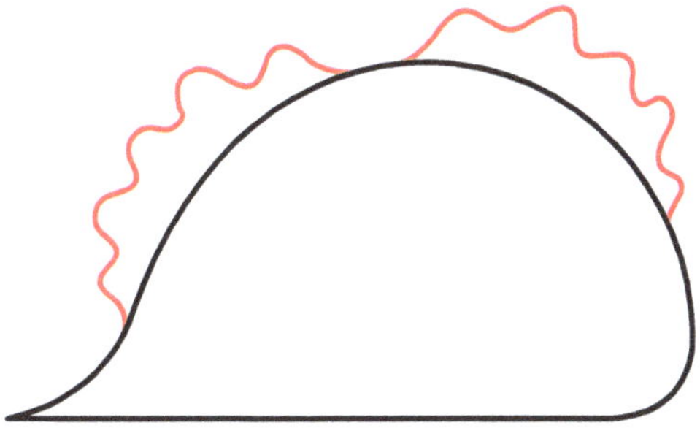

Add some frilly lettuce.

3

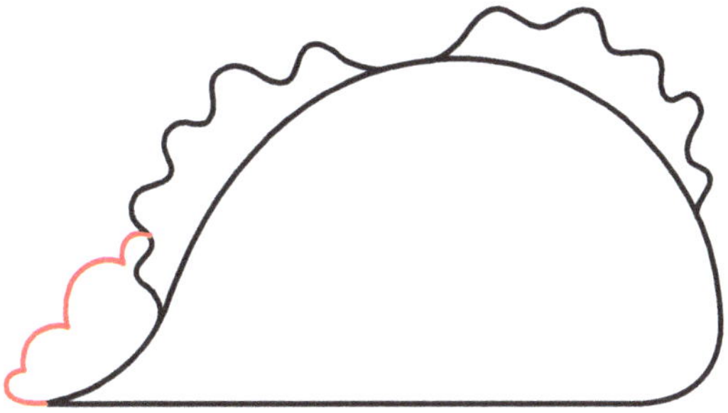

Add some meat, fish, or beans.

4

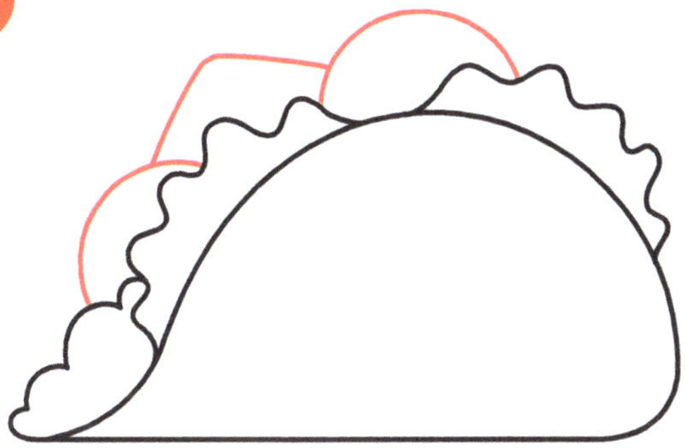

Now some extra toppings!

5

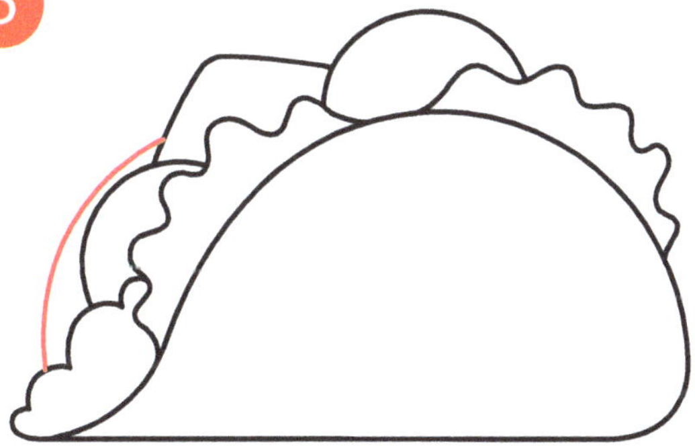

6

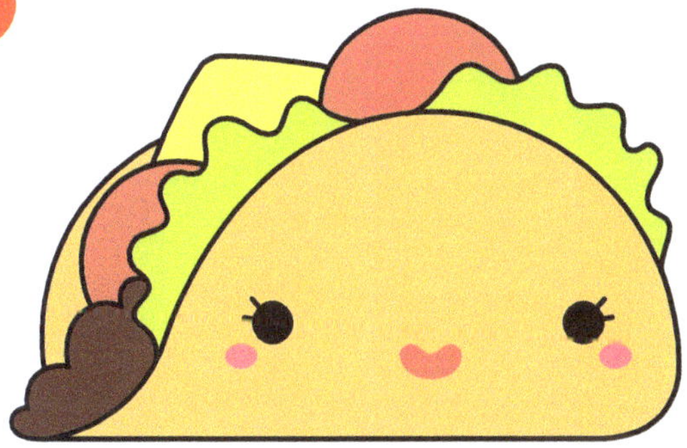

Looks tasty!

BLUSHING PIG

Shy pigs turn the pinkest pink!

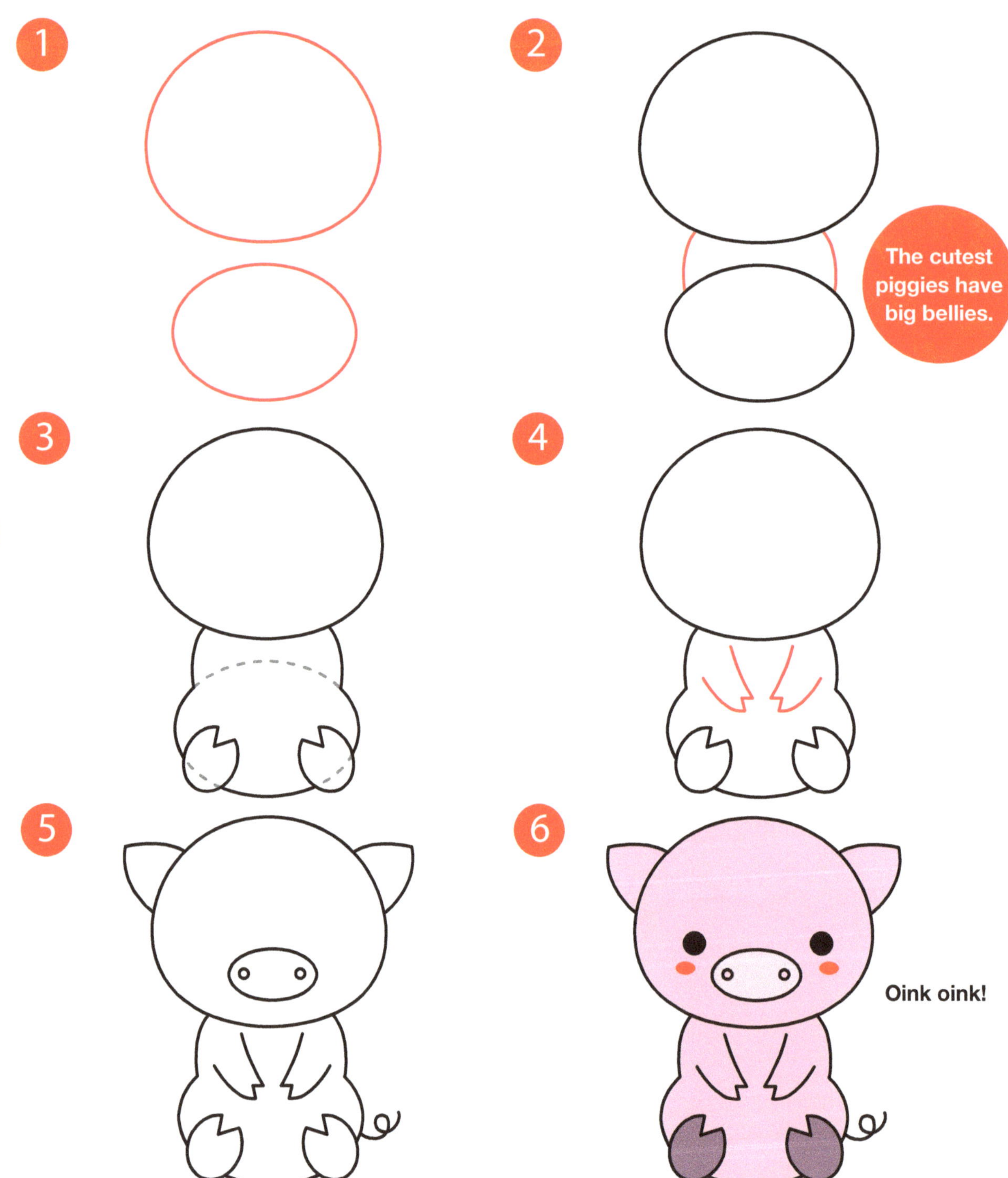

CHEESEBURGER

It's kawaii cuteness in a bun!

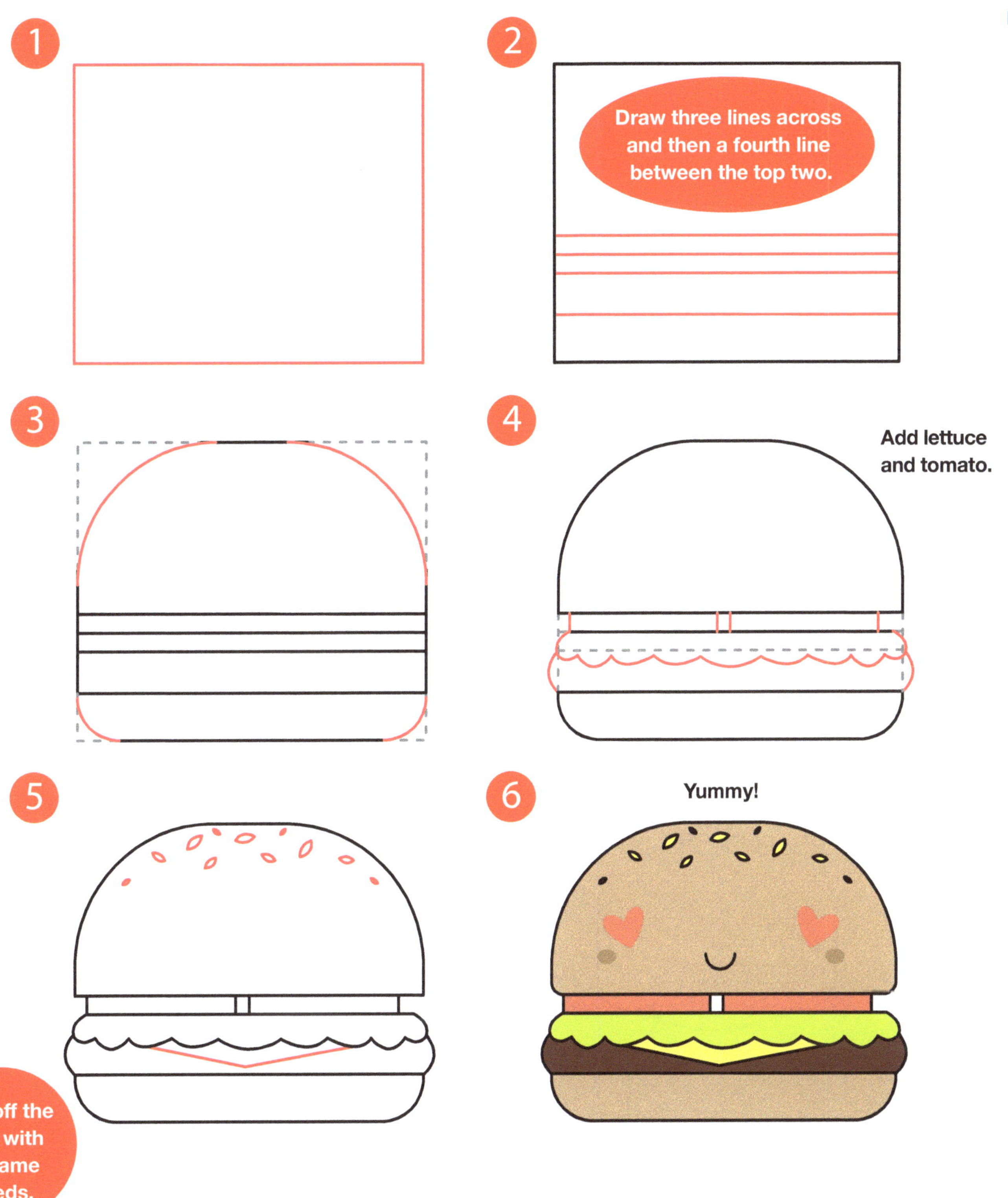

Top off the bun with sesame seeds.

HAPPY HAMSTER

Draw a pet hamster and then doodle him some snacks.

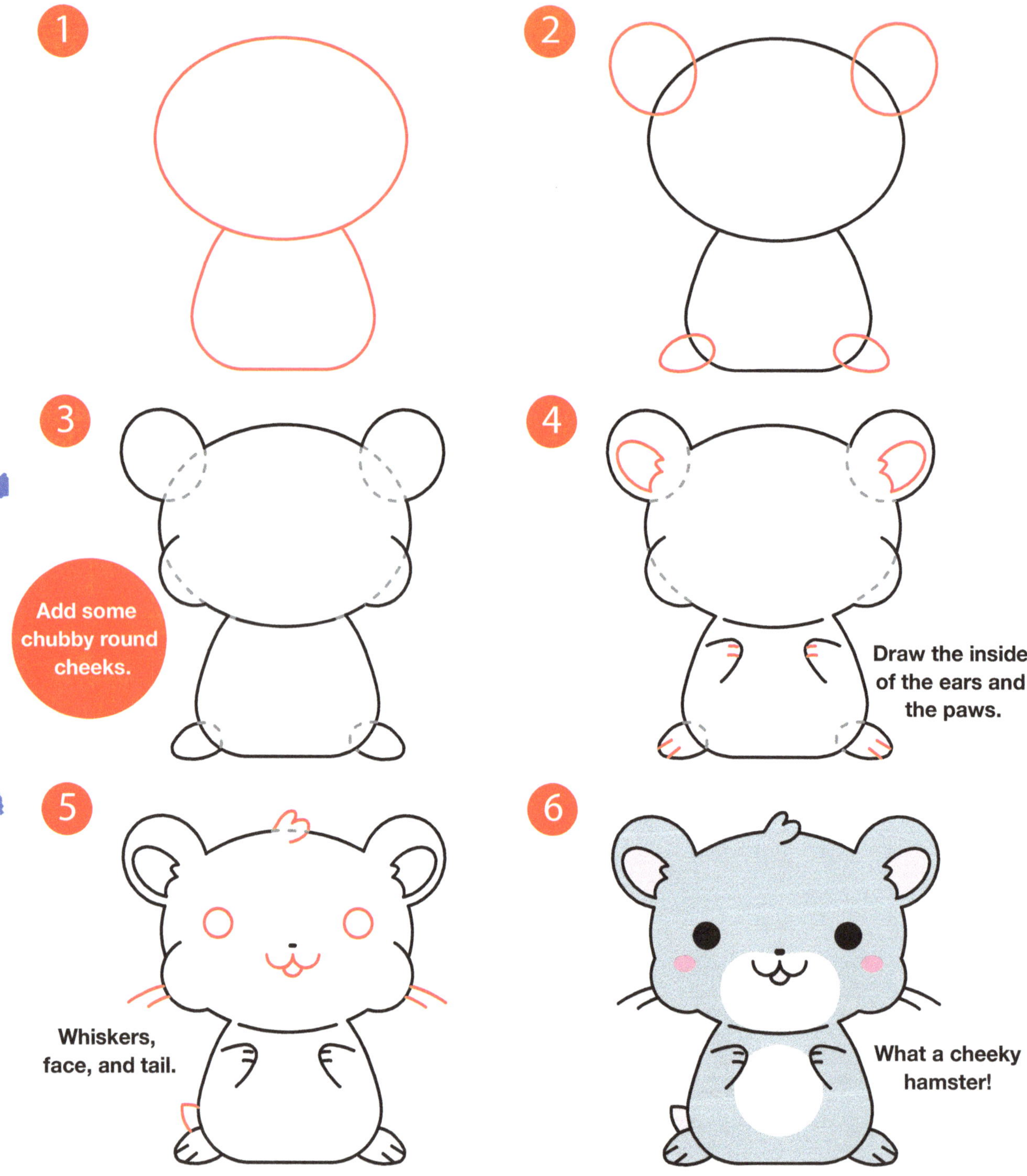

KAWAII CACTUS FUN

Create a cactus that prickles your fancy.

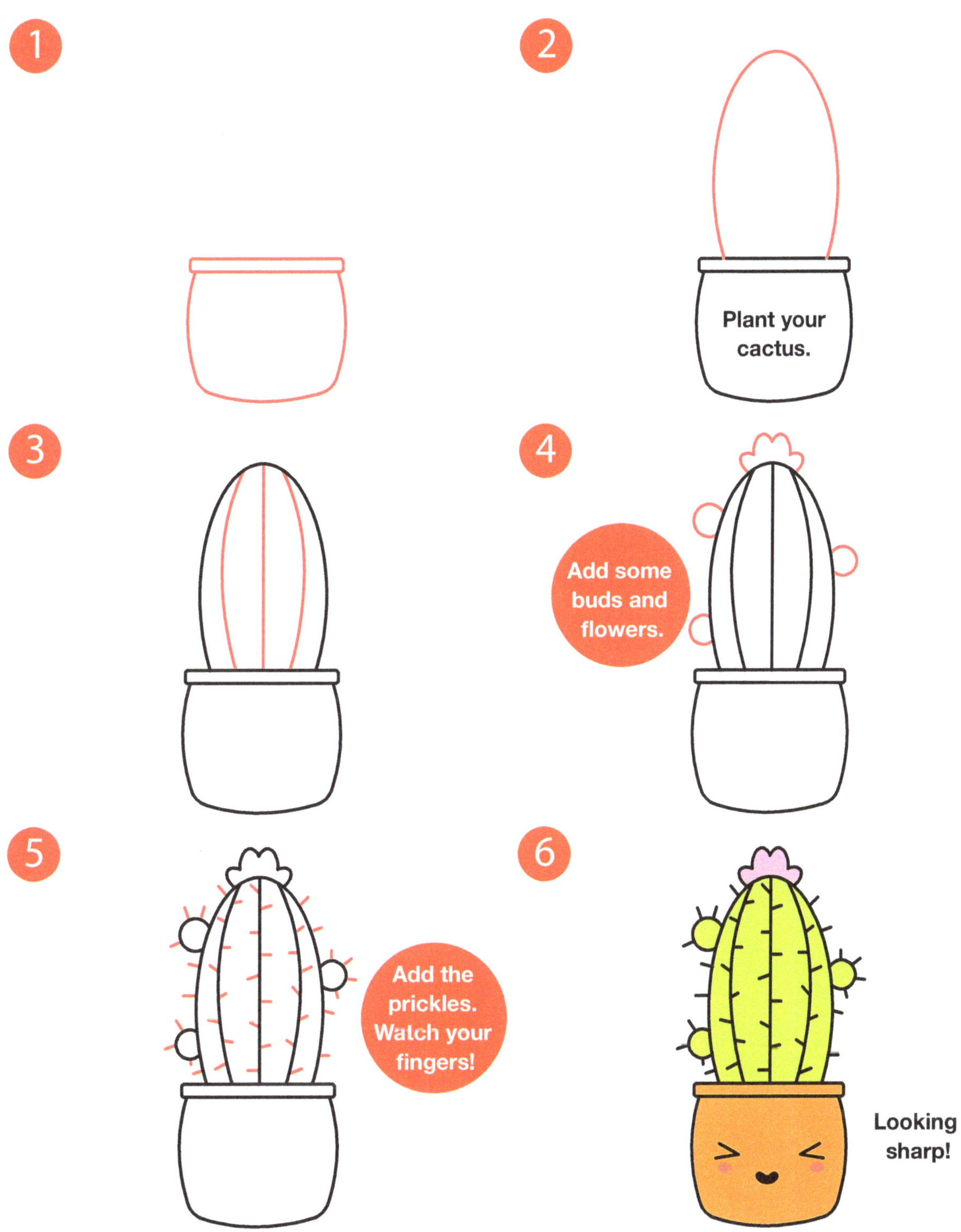

PENGUIN CHICK

Chill with a kawaii penguin!

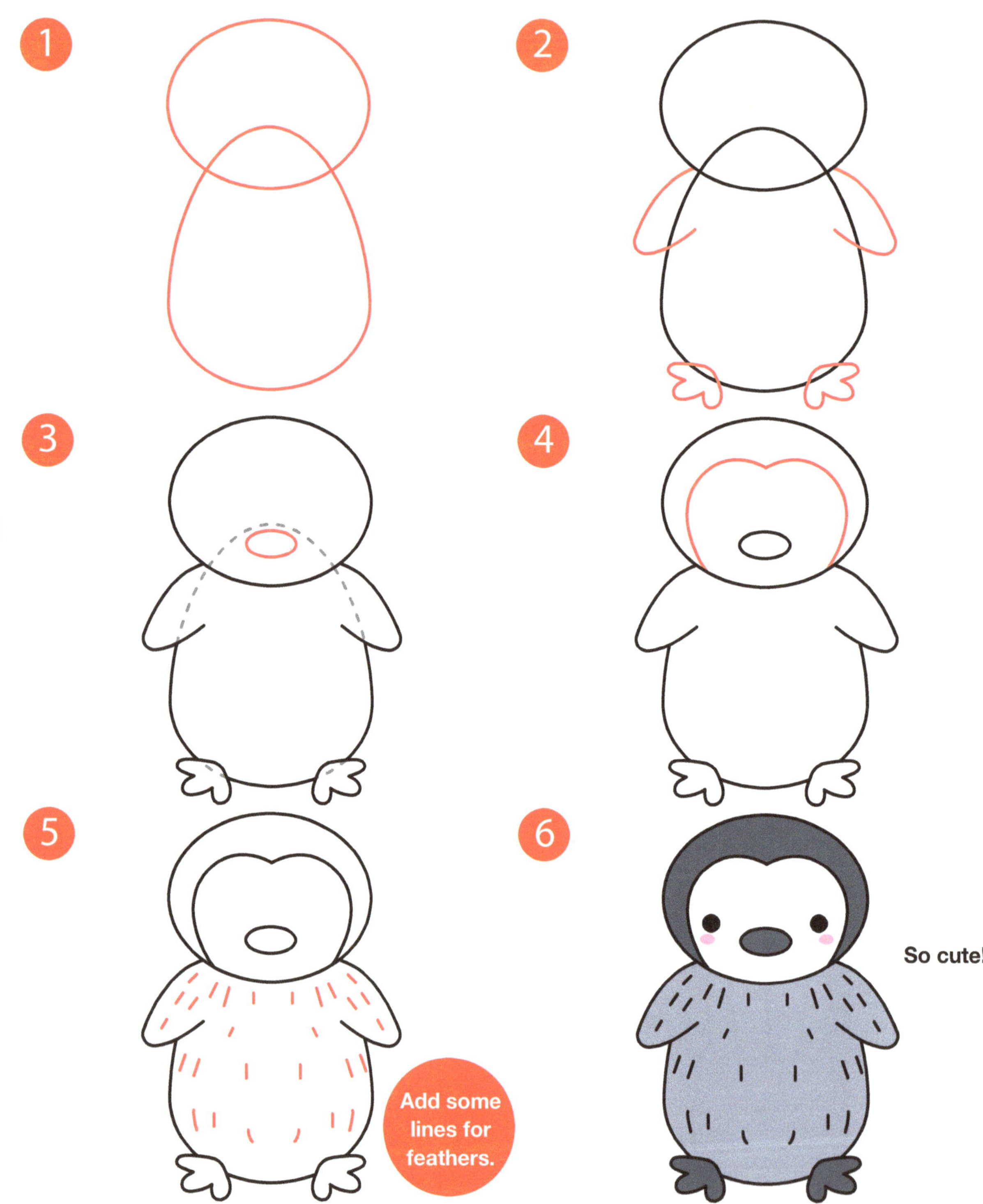

ICE CREAM CONE

Love ice cream? We sherbet you do!

1

2

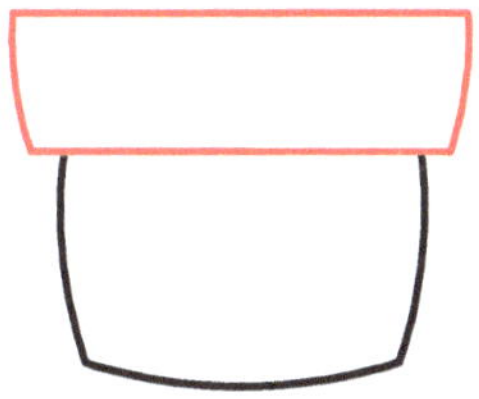

3

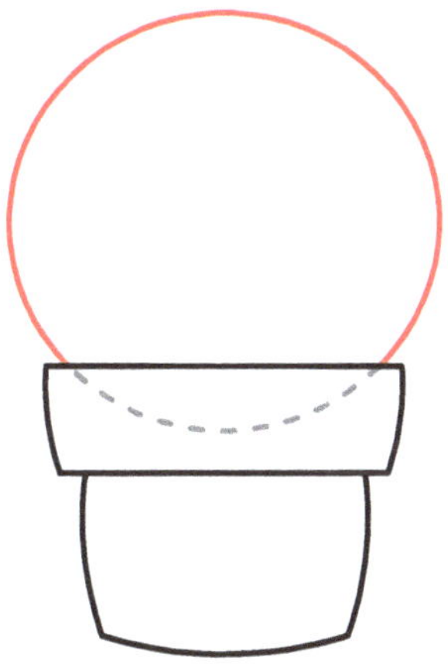

4

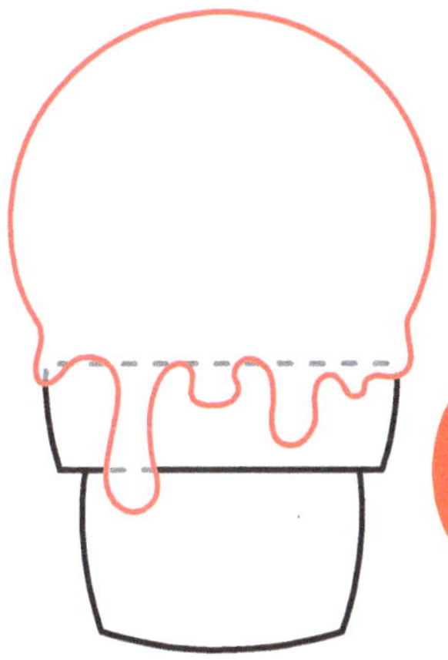

Add some drips for the melted ice cream.

5

Add the waffle texture and your favorite toppings!

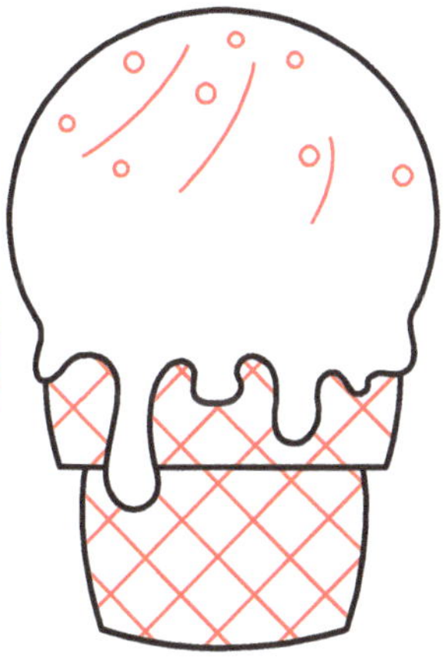

6

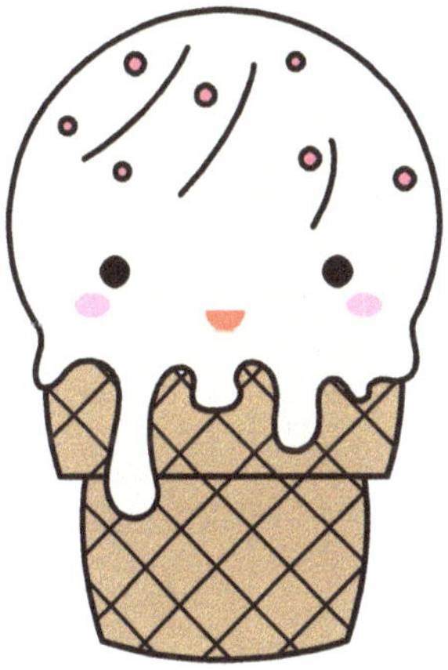

Cone-gratulations!

SUPER CUTE HERO

Summon your super drawing powers for this character!

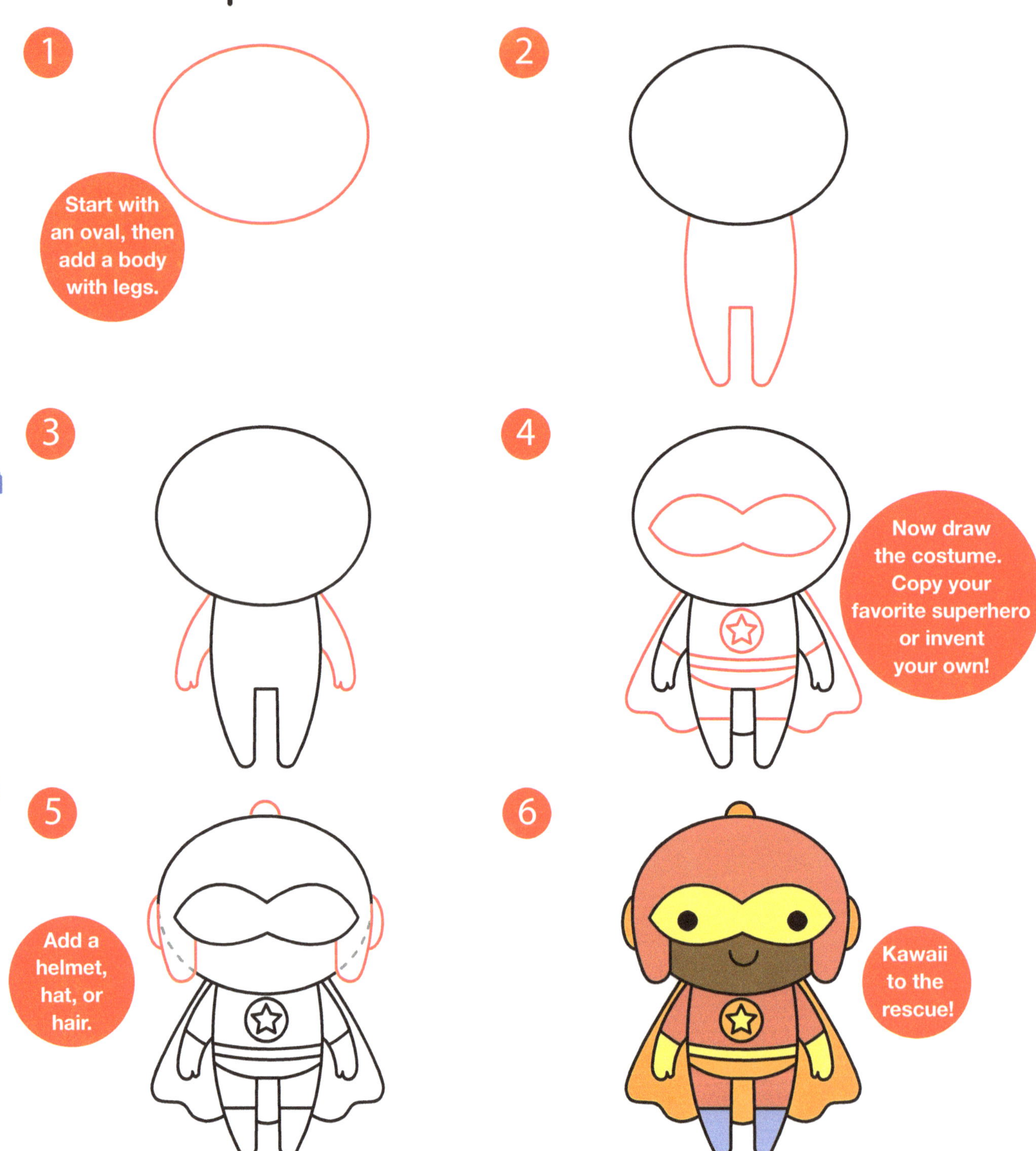

Part 3

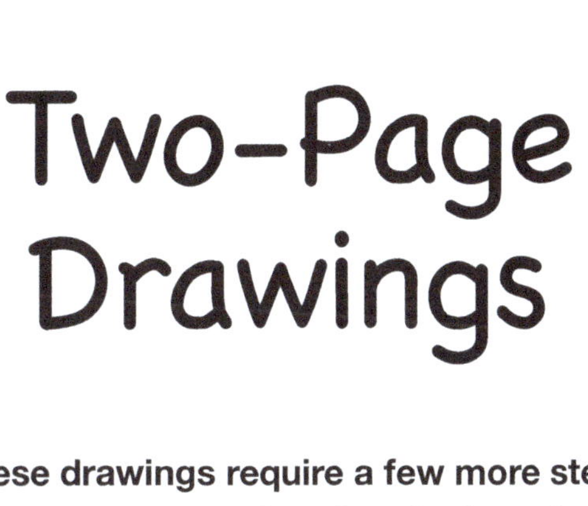

Two-Page Drawings

These drawings require a few more steps than the drawings you've already done, but that doesn't mean they are more difficult. Use the skills you learned while doing the one-step drawings, and don't forget to work lightly so you can erase your guidelines once your drawings are complete. Once you're done, trace super-cute versions of your favorite animals, people, food, or objects, to strengthen your keen kawaii skills.

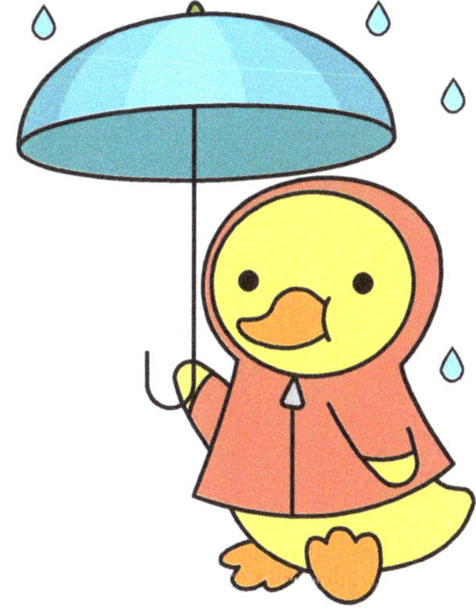

RAINY DAY DUCK

Ducks love to splash about on a rainy day.

1

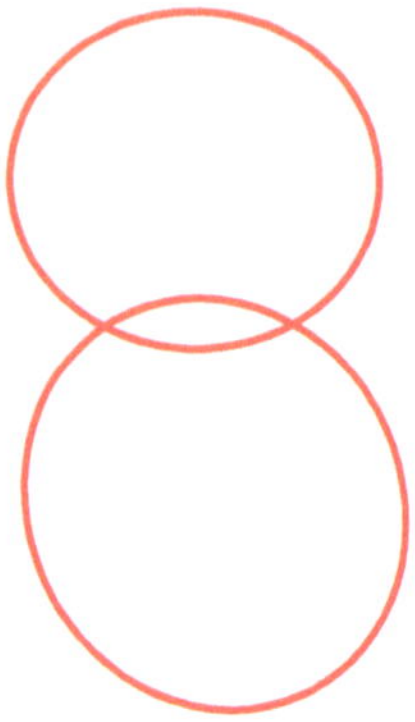

2

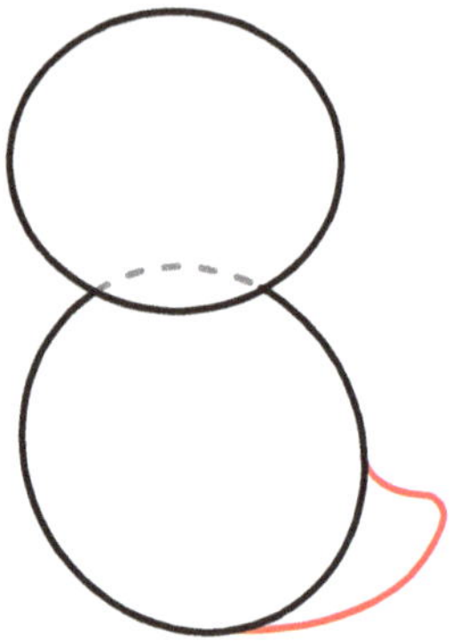

3

Add a hood.

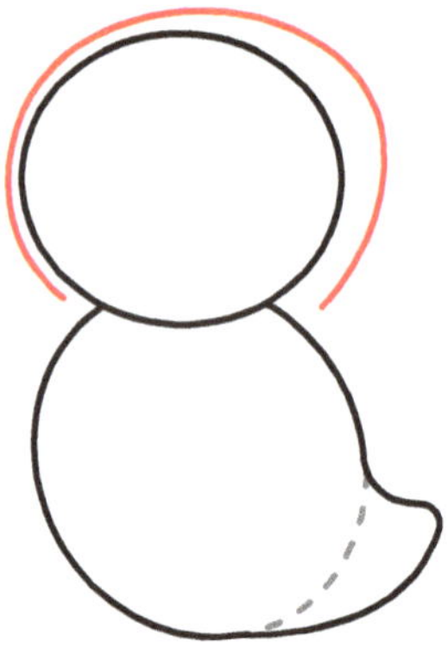

4

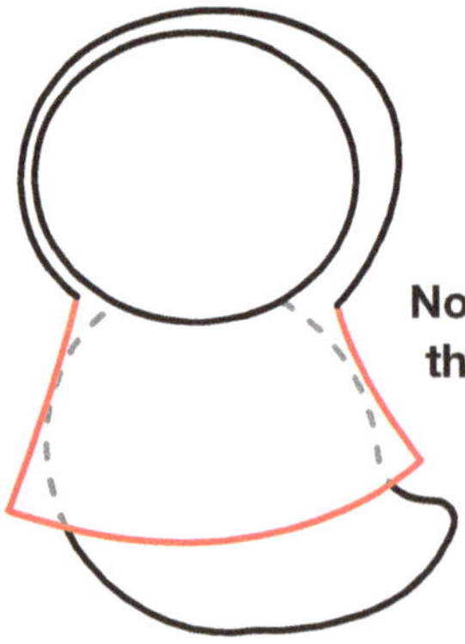

Now draw the cape.

5

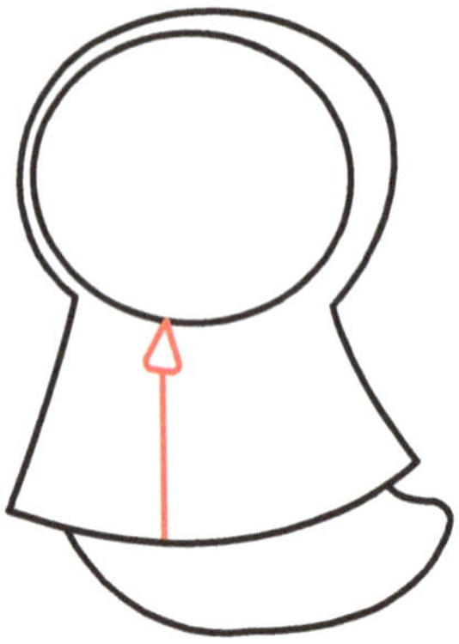

6

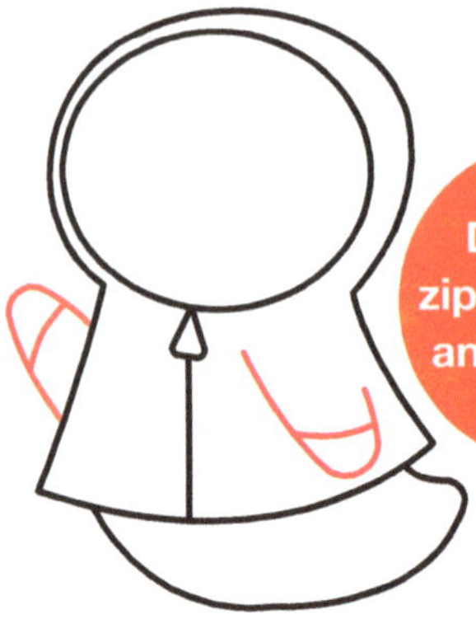

Draw the zipper, wings, and sleeves.

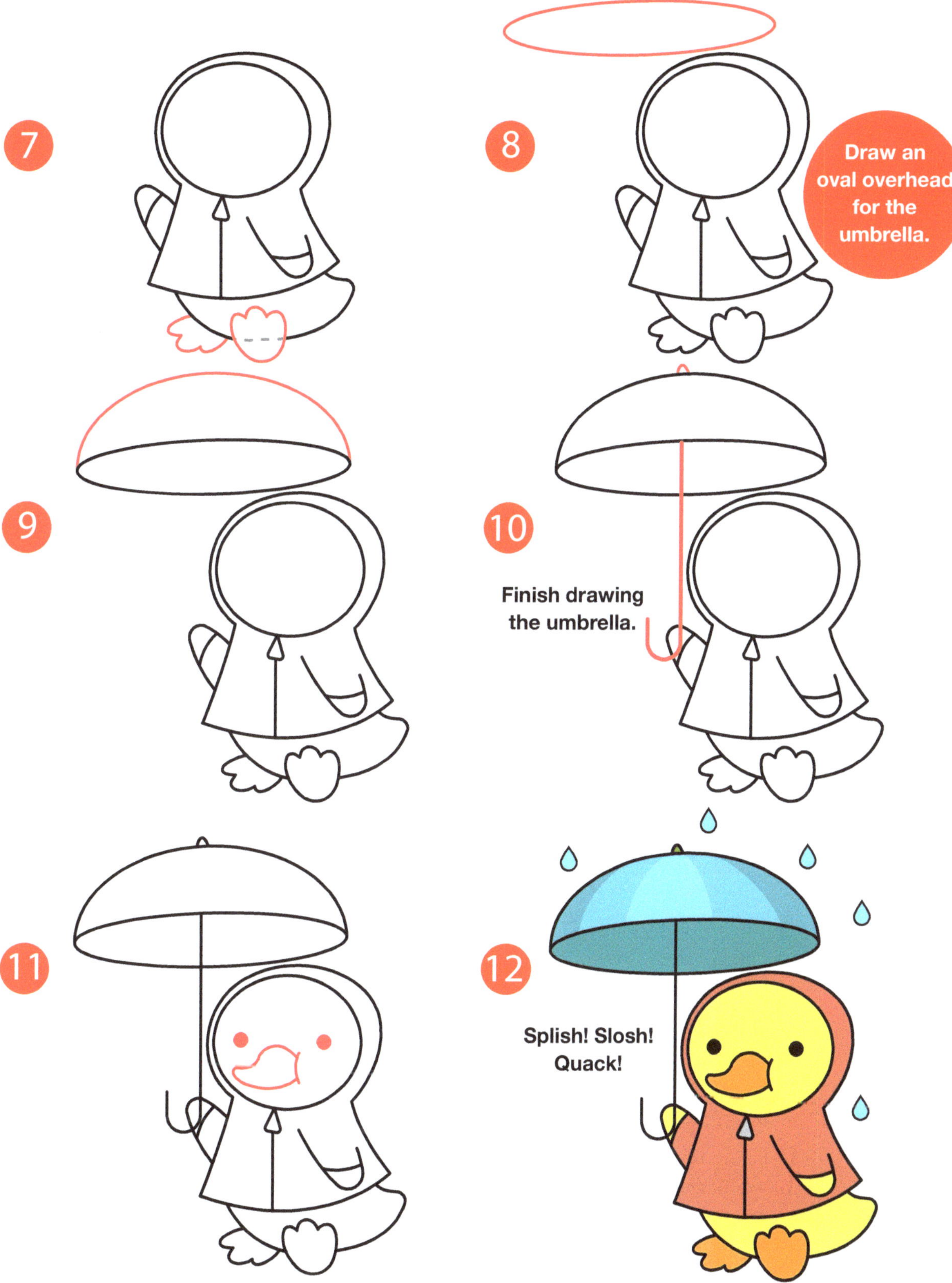
7
8
Draw an oval overhead for the umbrella.
9
10
Finish drawing the umbrella.
11
12
Splish! Slosh! Quack!

ICE CREAM SUNDAE

A tasty treat for any day of the week!

1 2

3 4

5 6

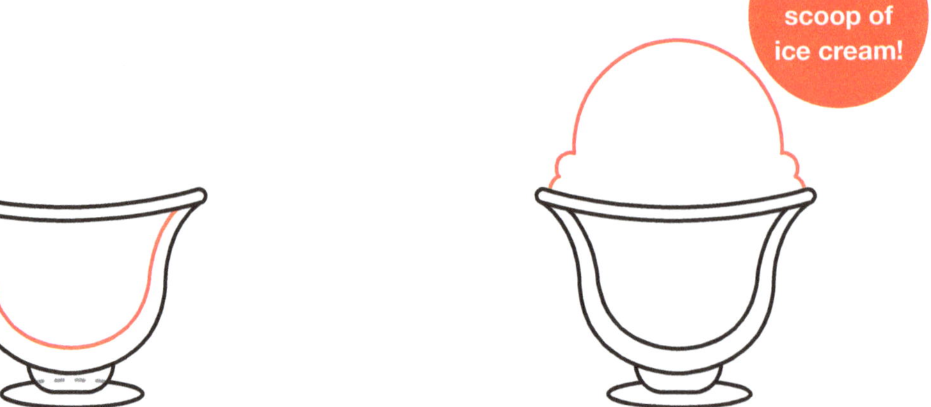

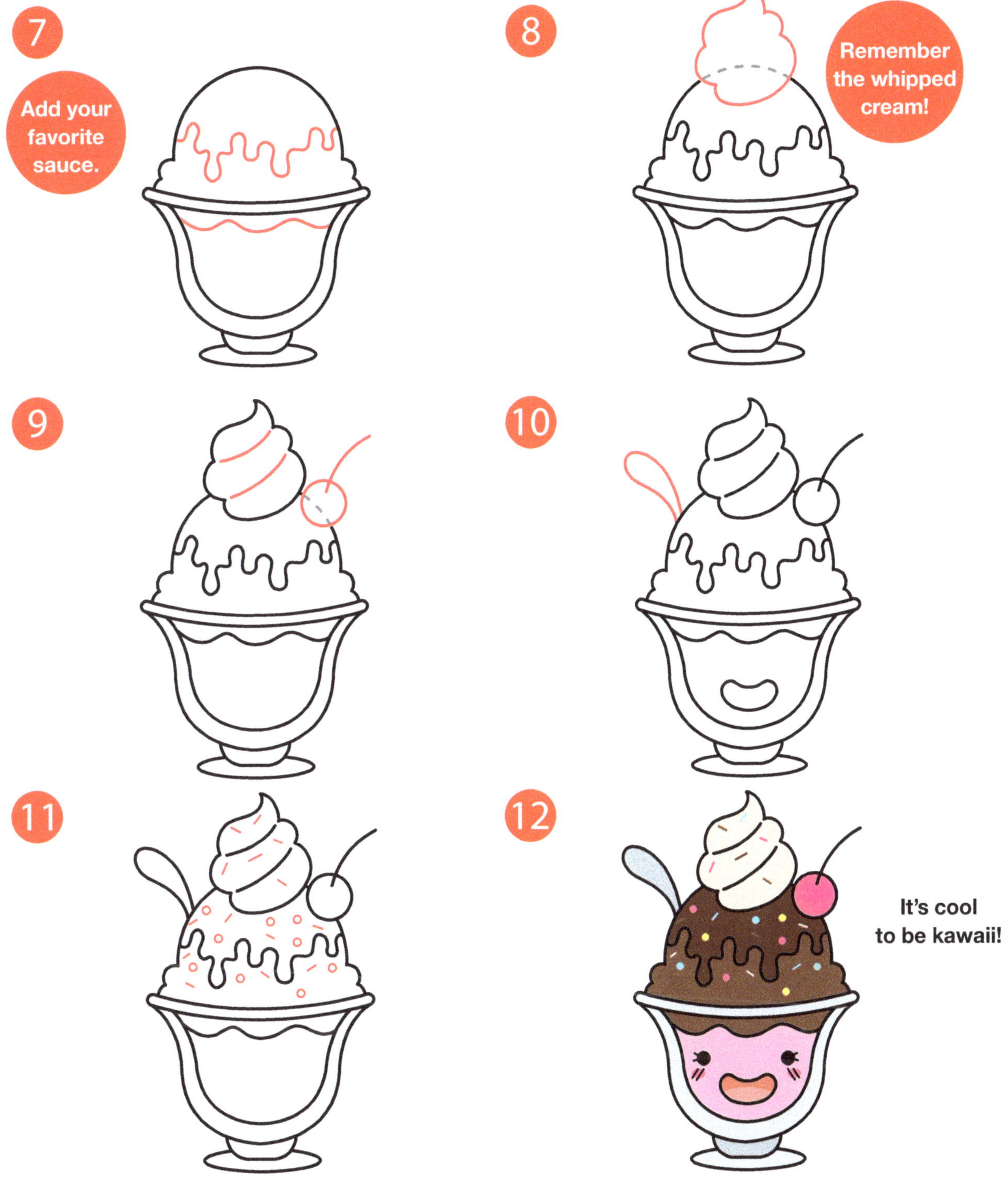
7
Add your favorite sauce.
8
Remember the whipped cream!
9
10
11
12
It's cool to be kawaii!
Now decorate!

TRY TRACING

Trace these kawaii characters to practice your skills.

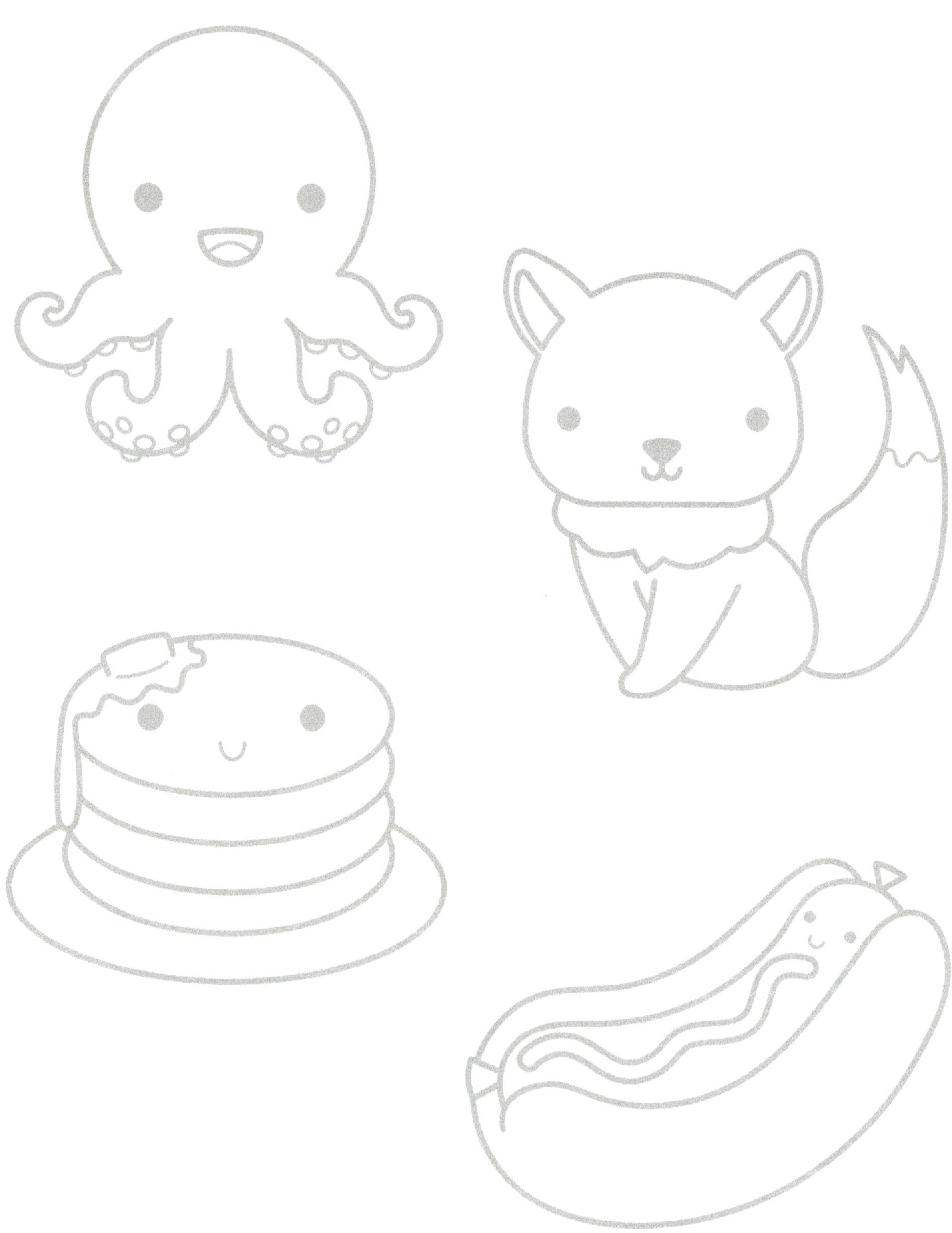

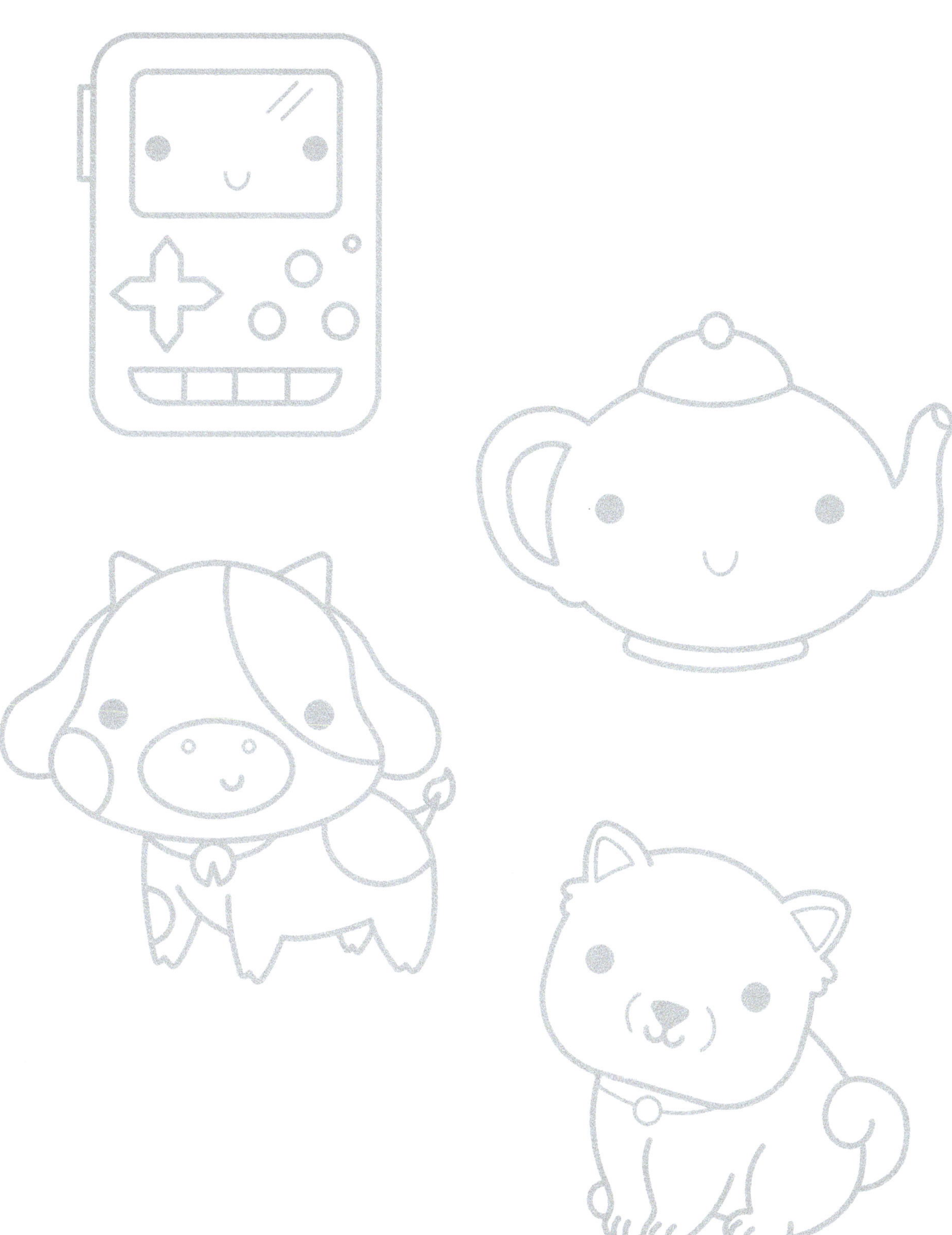

Part 4

Creative Exploration

Now it's time to get more creative! You've learned, step-by-step, how to draw cute creations and have also practiced your tracing. In this section, you can use fun backgrounds to stage your cute characters in different settings. Grab a pencil or pen and use your imagination!

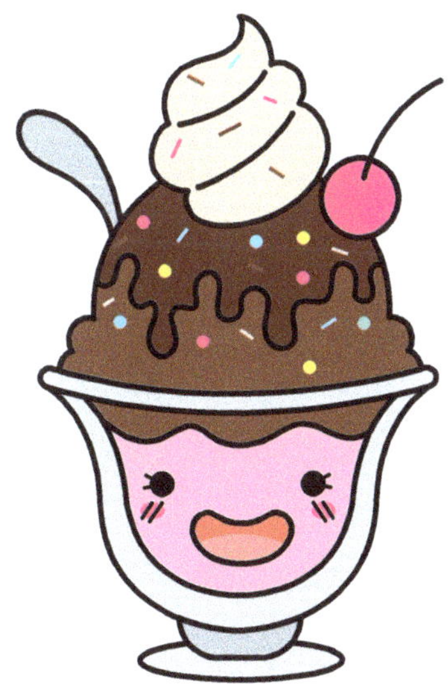

DECORATED SCENES

Draw your favorite kawaii characters in these different scenes.

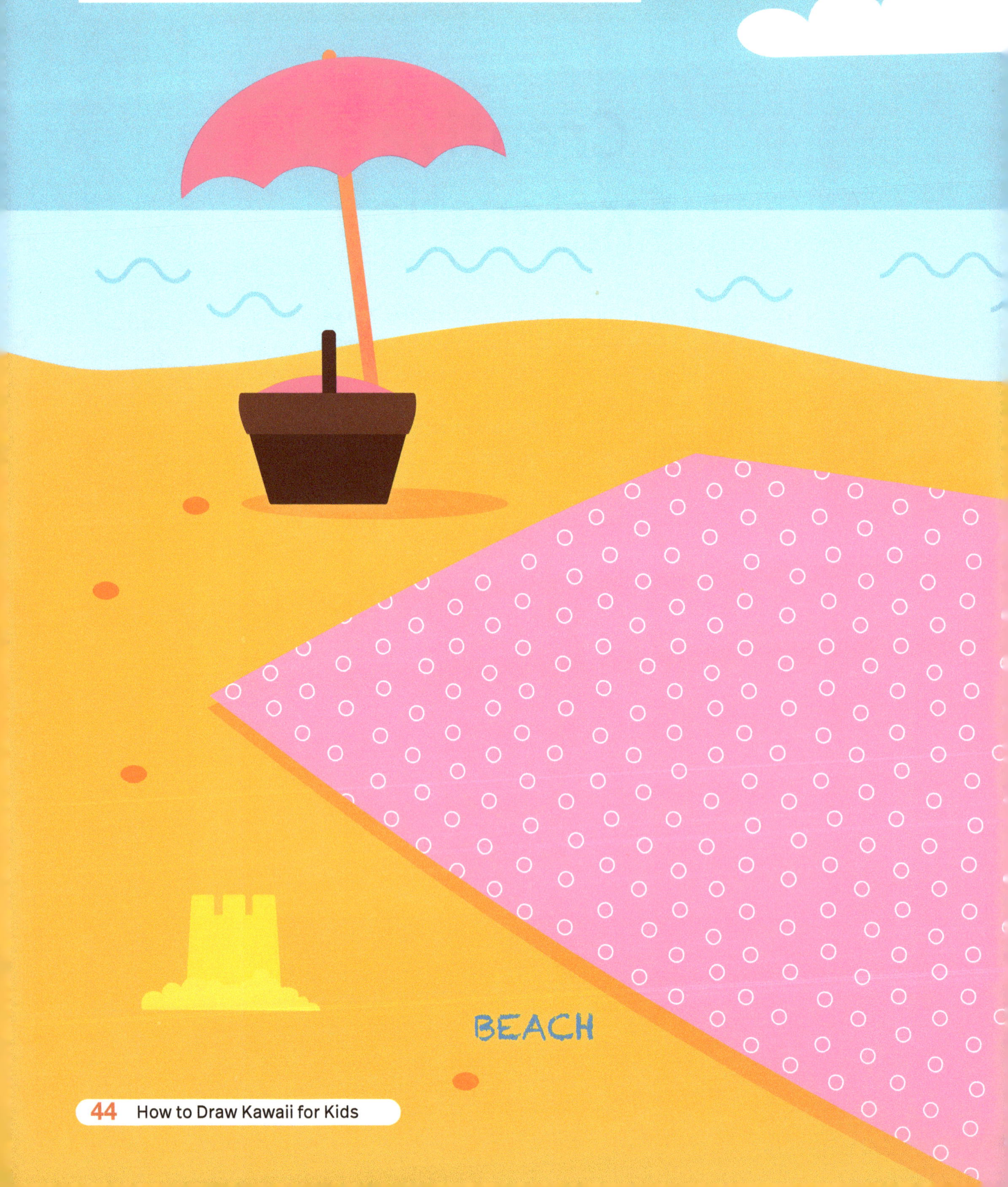

BEACH

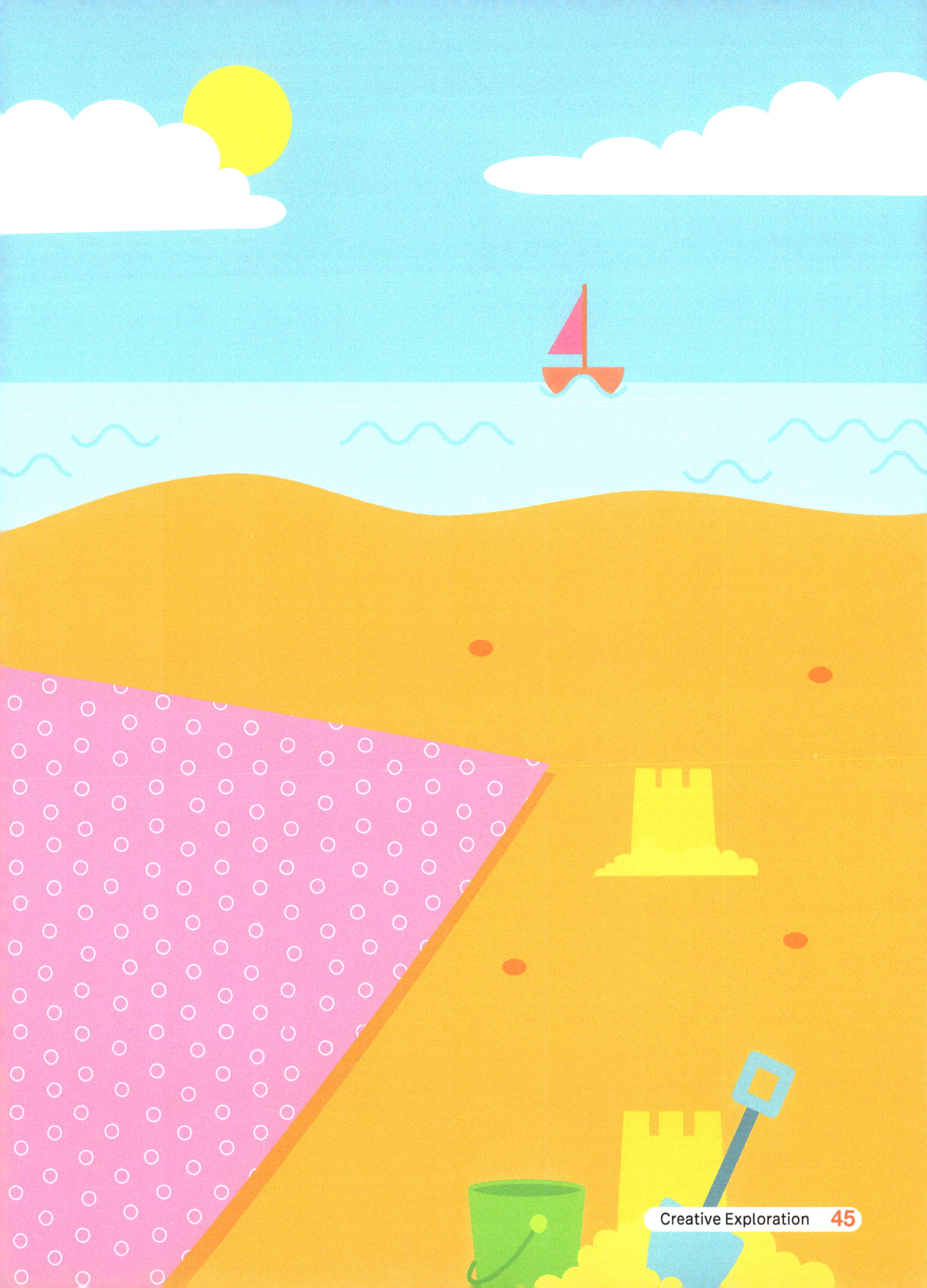

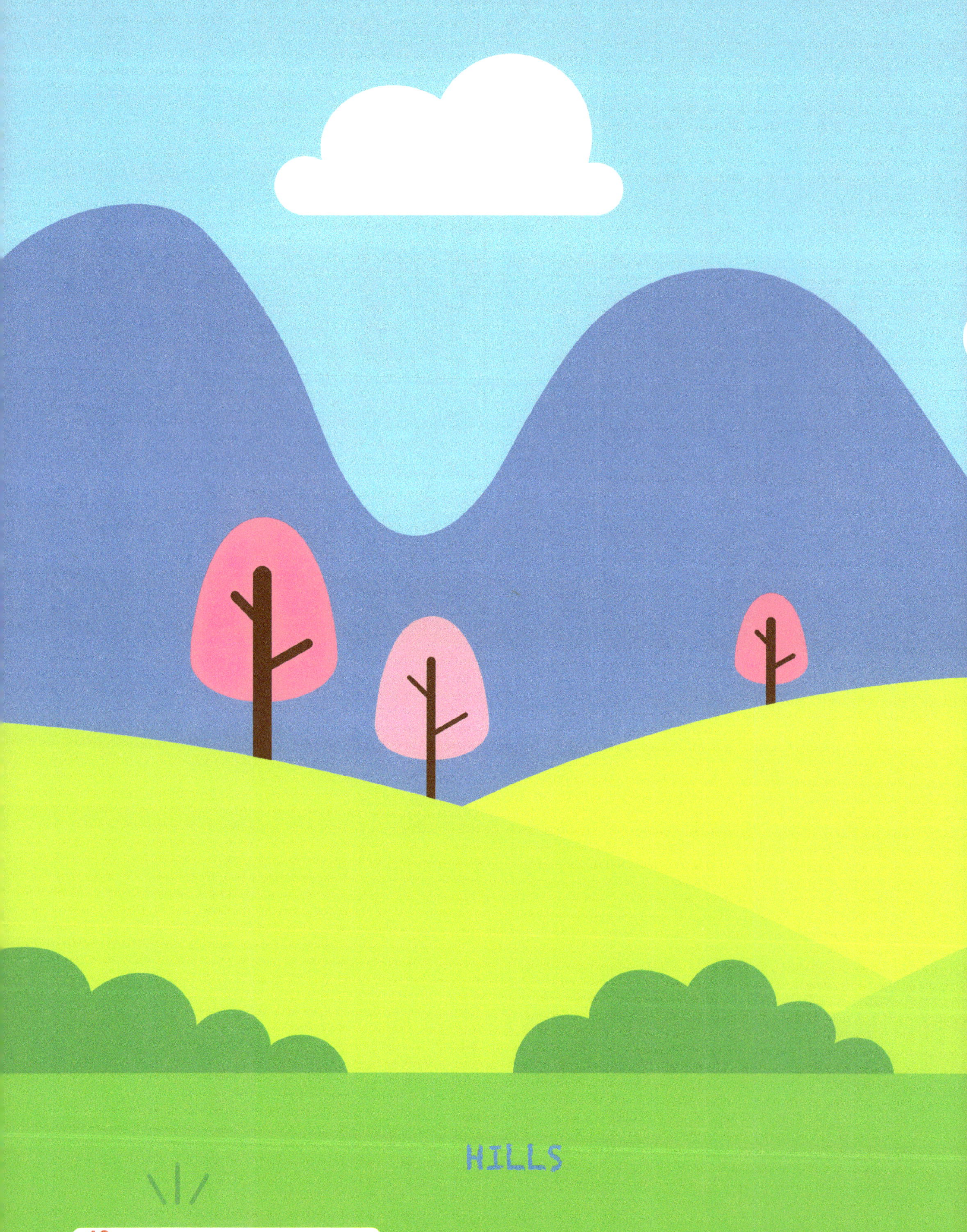
HILLS

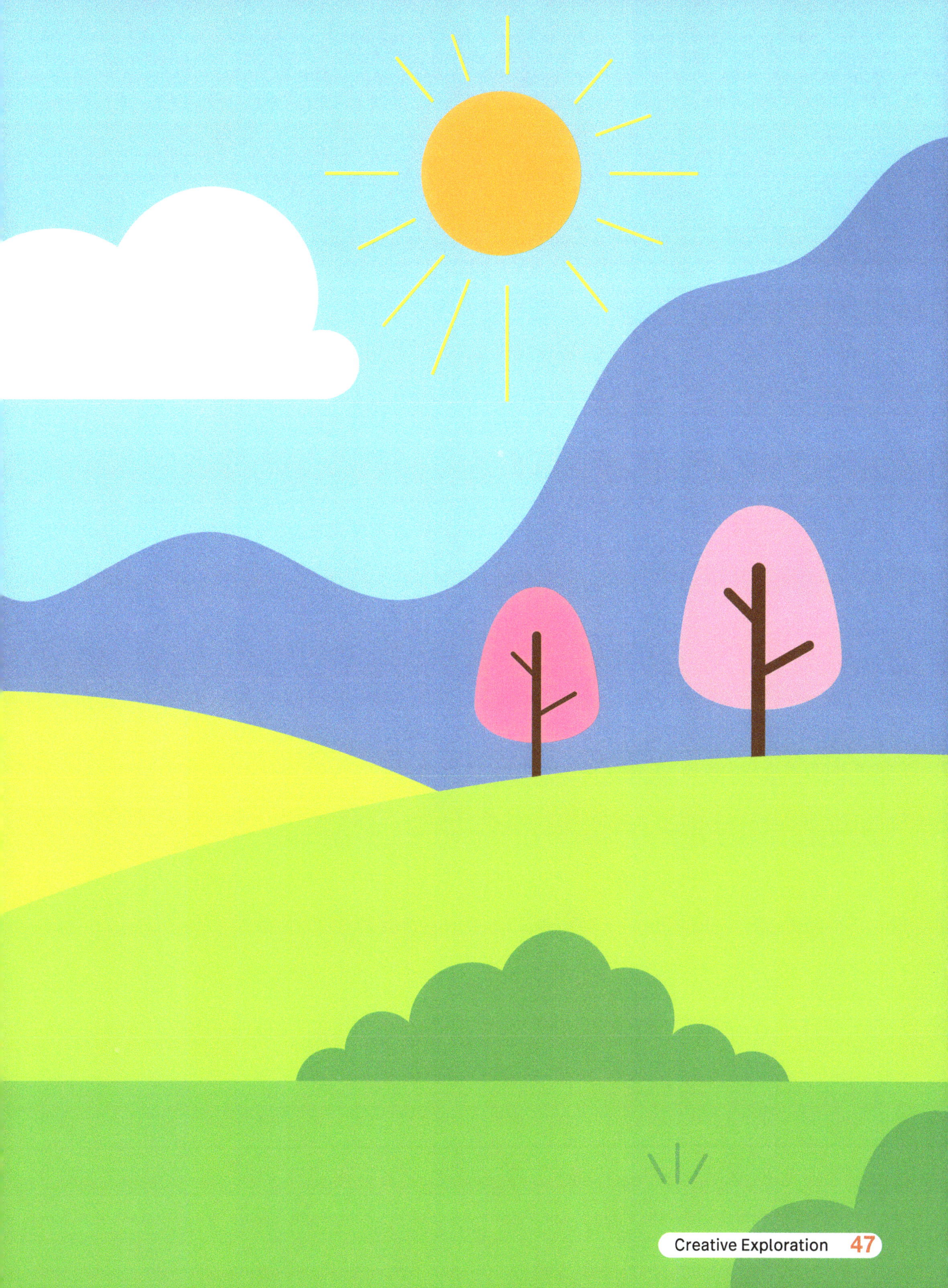

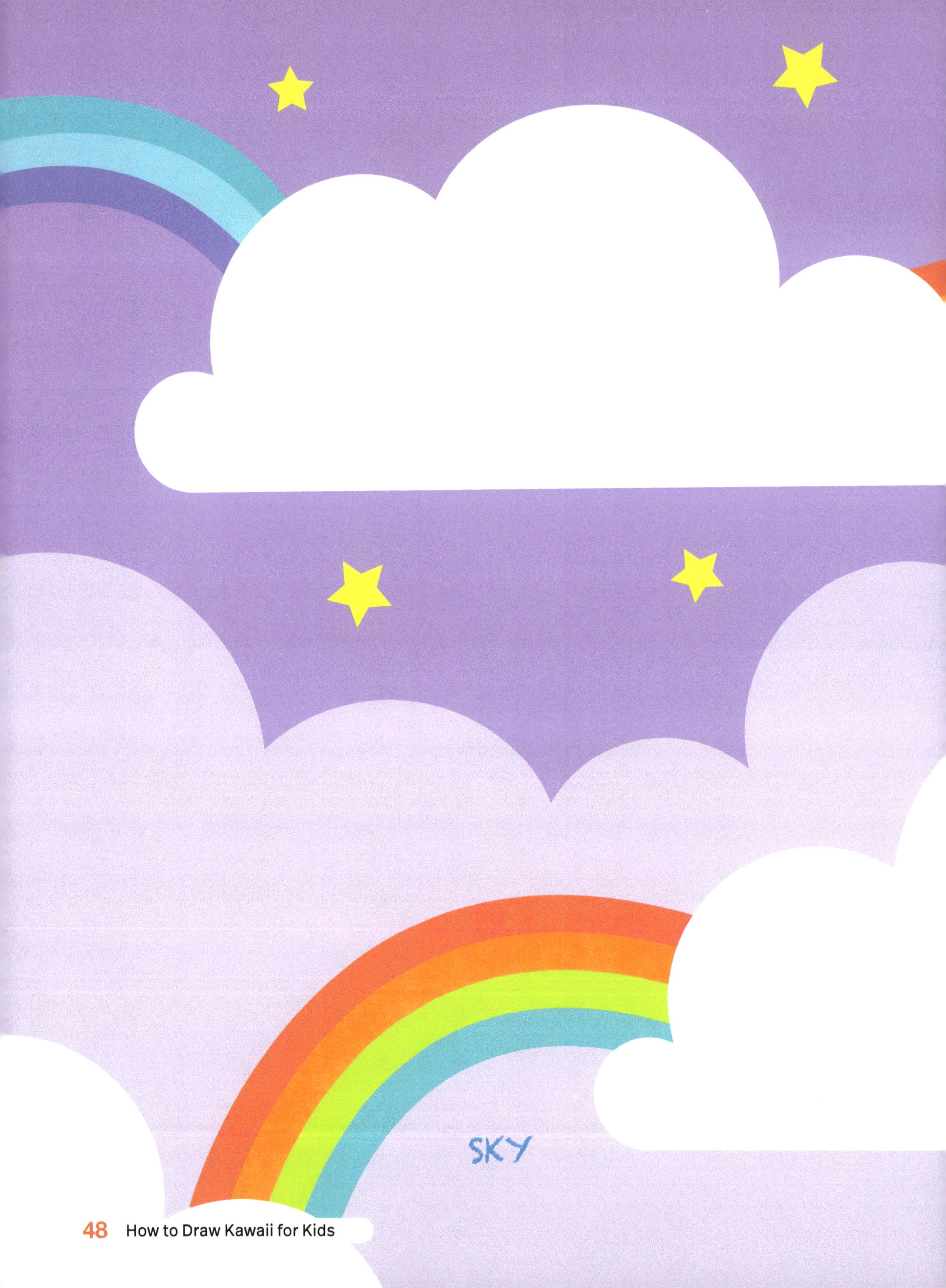
SKY

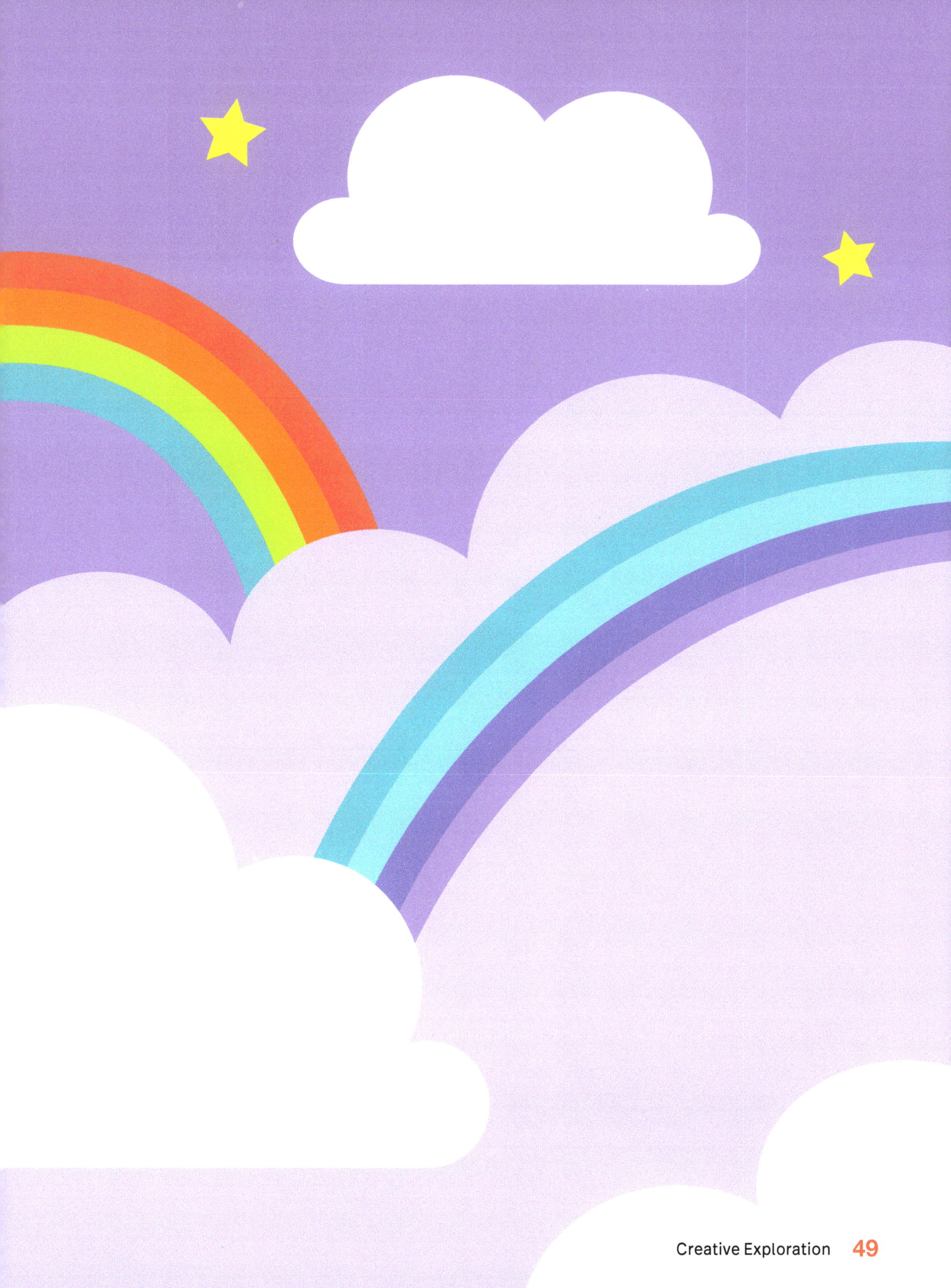

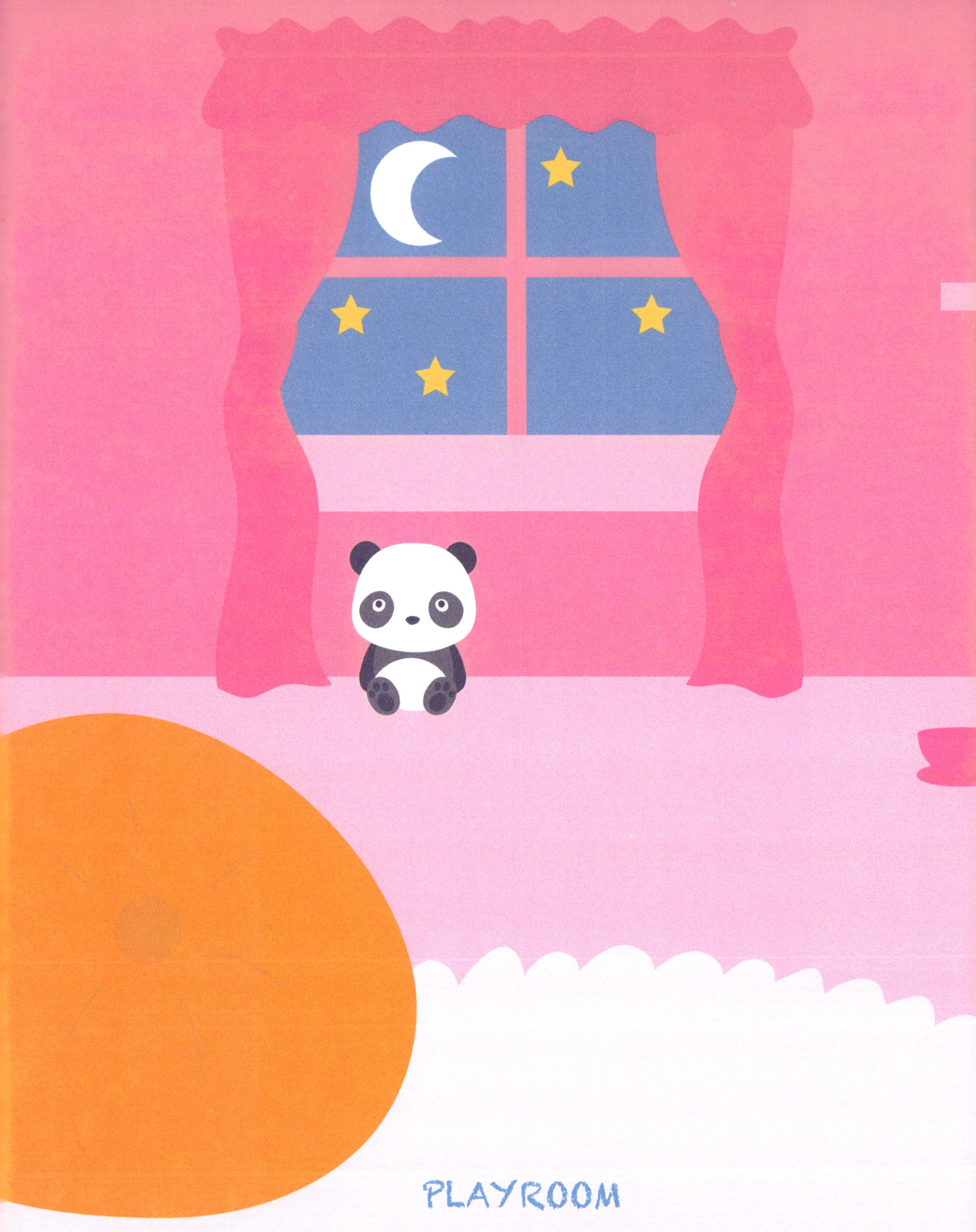

PLAYROOM

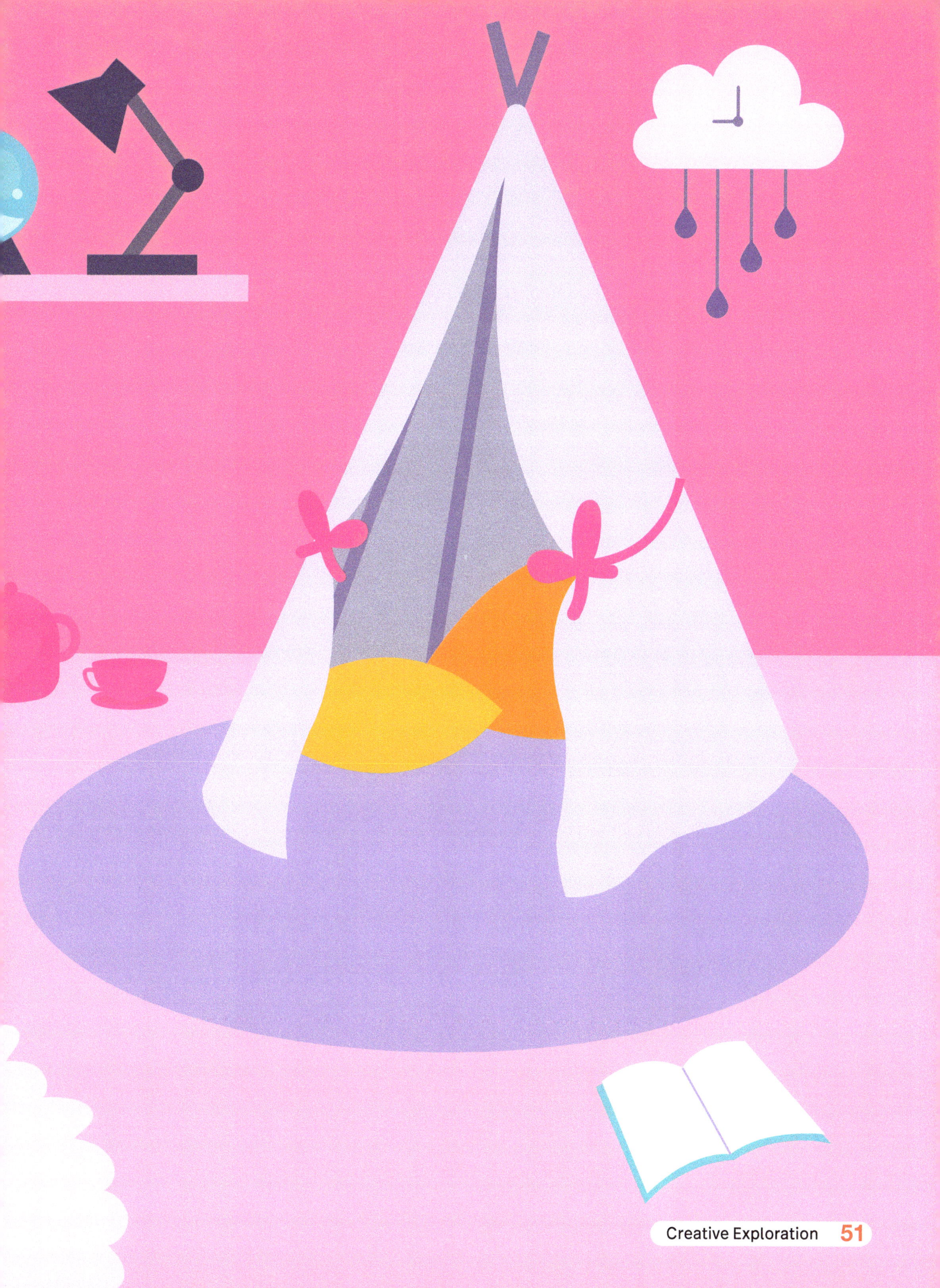

DRAWING PROMPTS

Now it's your turn to draw different kawaii characters the way you want them to look! Grab a piece of paper and draw from the following prompts.

→ Draw a family of peas in a pod.

→ Draw a unicorn galloping on a rainbow.

→ Draw a panda dressed as a cheerleader.

→ Draw your favorite sleepover snack.

→ Draw a penguin on a trampoline.

→ Draw a gang of different colored cats.

→ Draw a caramel milkshake.

→ Draw a houseplant in a pretty pot.

→ Draw yourself as a kawaii character!

→ Draw something you wish you had right now.